W9-AXM-107

THE

Men'sHealth

BIG MUSCLE
TRAINING
MANUAL

THE
Men'sHealth
BIG MUSCLE TRAINING MANUAL

SHED YOUR BELLY & BUILD YOUR BEST BODY FAST!

BY THE EDITORS OF *MEN'S HEALTH*

RODALE

The information in this book is meant to supplement, not replace, proper exercise training. All forms of exercise pose some inherent risks. The editors and publisher advise readers to take full responsibility for their safety and know their limits. Before practicing the exercises in this book, be sure that your equipment is well-maintained, and do not take risks beyond your level of experience, aptitude, training, and fitness. The exercise and dietary programs in this book are not intended as a substitute for any exercise routine or dietary regimen that may have been prescribed by your doctor. As with all exercise and dietary programs, you should get your doctor's approval before beginning.

Mention of specific companies, organizations, or authorities in this book does not imply endorsement by the author or publisher, nor does mention of specific companies, organizations, or authorities imply that they endorse this book, its author, or the publisher.

Internet addresses and telephone numbers given in this book were accurate at the time it went to press.

© 2013 by Rodale Inc.

All rights reserved. No part of this publication may be reproduced or transmitted in any form or by any means, electronic or mechanical, including photocopying, recording, or any other information storage and retrieval system, without the written permission of the publisher.

Men's Health is a registered trademark of Rodale Inc.

Printed in the United States of America
Rodale Inc. makes every effort to use acid-free ⊛, recycled paper ♲.

Part opener photos and photos on pages 21, 51, 113, 153, and 173 by Scott McDermott
Exercise pose photos by Beth Bischoff, except walking pushup photos on page 159 by John Hamel
Illustration on page 4 by Scott Holladay
Photos on pages 12, 13, and 29 by Darryl Estine
Page 18 photo/illustration: photo by Darryl Estrine and illustration by Molly Borman
Equipment photos on pages 32 and 33 by Levi Brown

Book design by Mark Michaelson

Library of Congress Cataloging-in-Publication Data is on file with the publisher.

ISBN 978–1–60961–999–2

Distributed to the trade by Macmillan

2 4 6 8 10 9 7 5 3   paperback

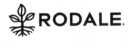

We inspire and enable people to improve their lives and the world around them.

rodalebooks.com

CONTENTS

INTRODUCTION

What you want.

What you need.

Two very different things. But right here, right now, as you hold this book in your hands, you cannot have one without the other.

What you want—what you've *always* wanted—is a lean, strong body. You want bigger muscles, but you also want functional strength. You want power, explosiveness, and panther-smoothness in every move. You want the kind of body that lets you cruise through not just the everyday tasks, but the weekend log-splitting and couch-moving sessions (because, hey, we're at our best when we're of use). You want to play better at everything. You want stares. You want to cut a swath at work. You want to carry your best girl up a flight of stairs.

You want to dominate your day.

Too many guys squeak through their days. Is that you? You know the type—they have sore knees, biting lower backs, and a growing paunch. They have caffeine headaches, feet of clay, and a dead furnace in the heart of their soul. That's the trap for men, isn't it?

The temptation: Be that faux mover and shaker like those old school guys, fill your day with work and food and cut loose when the sun goes down. But it's a sucker play. Next thing you know, years have passed and you're on your way to becoming . . . like all those other achy, tired men who think they're far more than they really are.

Yeah, we know what you want.

But let's talk about what you need.

A plan. Some motivation. Some balls. You see, most men forget that achieving what you want requires movement. You want happiness? Happiness is a choice. Happiness takes guts. If it didn't, everyone would look and feel the way they want. They don't.

You can.

And you will. Because *The Men's Health Big Muscle Training Manual* contains everything a motivated man needs to get what he wants.

You need knowledge. From how muscle works to the biomechanics of your body to what it takes to build a better human male, this book is packed with guidance and science. All you have to do is read and execute.

You need workouts. No matter what your fitness level, there are enough workouts in here to transform the male cast of *The Big Bang Theory* into the cast of *The Expendables*. (That's a movie we'd like to see, by the way).

You need food. The chapters on eating will fuel your feasts with intelligent meals, snacks, and body-boosting nutrition. We mean the following statement both literally and figuratively: *No man should ever eat crap.*

You need progression. As you gain, you need new challenges. The workouts in this book get stronger as you do. Their plateau-busting powers are built-in. With every burn, every rep, every sweat-silhouette left on every workout bench, you'll know you're achieving everything you want.

You need . . . you. The whole thing really comes down to one question: Will you be a friend to yourself? Or a lifelong shoulder-shrugger?

You know what you want.

You have everything you need.

Go forth. Sweat out the old you. Carve the new you from a block of oak. Make the choice.

Dominate your day.

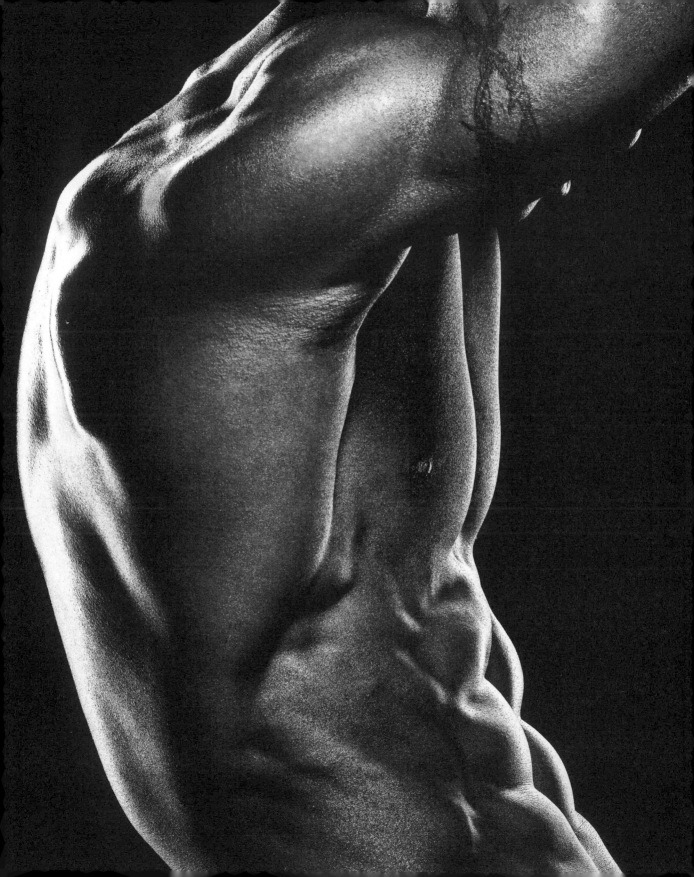

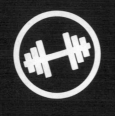

PART ONE

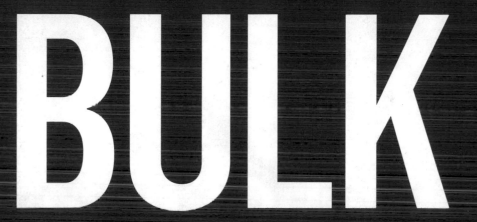

EVERYTHING YOU
NEED TO KNOW
TO BUILD MUSCLE
AND SHED FAT FAST

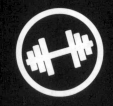

CHAPTER 1

MEET YOUR MYOFIBRILS

(OR, HOW YOUR BODY BUILDS MUSCLE)

What do you know about muscle?

Your body has about 650 of them. It doesn't matter that you care about only four or five muscles. You need every one in order to perform the normal functions of everyday life—eating, breathing, walking, holding in your stomach at the beach. Granted, you don't need to spend a lot of time thinking about most of your muscles. The 200 muscles involved in walking do the job whether you monitor them or not. You could try to impress your friends at parties by telling them the gluteus maximus is the body's strongest muscle, or that the latissimus dorsi (in your middle back) is the largest, or that a middle-ear muscle called the stapedius is the smallest. But it probably won't work, unless you have some really unusual friends. And muscle trivia can't capture the wonder of muscles themselves—the brilliance of coordinated muscles in motion, the magnificence of well-developed muscles in isolation. We hope, in the following chapter, to help you understand a little more about how your muscles work, and thus how to make them bigger, stronger, and more aesthetically pleasing. You can accomplish all three— quickly—if you know what's going on beneath the surface.

MUSCLE FIBERS HOLD THE SECRET

Your skeletal muscles—the ones you check out in the mirror—have two main types of fibers. Type I fibers, also called slow-twitch, are used mainly for endurance activities. Type II, or fast-twitch, begin to work when a task utilizes more than 25 percent of your maximum strength. A movement doesn't have to be "slow" for the slow-twitch fibers to take over; it just has to be an action that doesn't require much of your fast-twitch strength. And an effort doesn't have to be "fast" to call your fast-twitch fibers into play. A personal-record

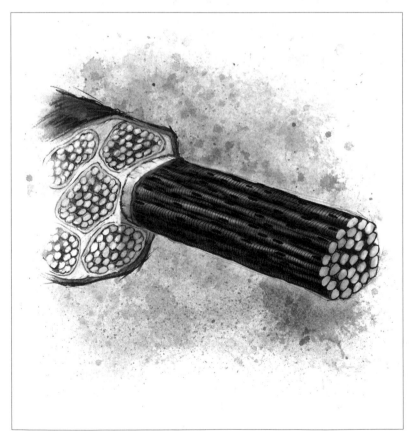

bench press is going to use every possible fast-twitch fiber (plus all the slow-twitchers, as we'll explain below), even though the bar probably isn't moving very fast.

Most people are thought to have a more or less equal mix of slow- and fast-twitch fibers. (Elite athletes are obvious exceptions—a gifted marathoner was probably born with more slow- than fast-twitch fibers, just as an Olympic-champion sprinter or NFL running back probably started life with more fast-twitch fibers.) However, the fast-twitch fibers are twice as big as the slow ones, with the potential to get even bigger. Slow-twitch fibers can get bigger, too, although not to the same extent. So one strategy comes immediately to mind. . . .

TO GROW LARGE, LIFT LARGE

When you begin a task, no matter if it's as simple as getting out of bed or as complex as swinging a golf club, your muscles operate on two basic principles of physiology:

1. The all-or-nothing principle states that either a muscle fiber gets into the action or it doesn't. (As Yoda said, long ago in a galaxy far away, "There is no try.") If it's in, it's all the way in. So when you get up to walk to the bathroom, incredibly enough, a small percentage of your muscle fibers are working as hard as they can to get you there. And, more important, all the other fibers are inactive.

2. The size principle requires that the smallest muscle fibers get into a task first. If the task—a biceps curl, for example—requires less than 25 percent of your biceps' strength, then the slow-twitch fibers will handle it by themselves. When the weight exceeds 25 percent of their strength, the type II, fast-twitch fibers jump in. The closer you get to the limits of your strength, the more fast-twitch fibers get involved.

Here's why this is important: One of the most pervasive myths in the muscle world is that merely exhausting a muscle will bring all its fibers into play. So, in theory, if you did a lot of repetitions with a light weight, eventually your biggest type II fibers would help out because the smaller fibers would be too tired to lift the weight. But the size principle tells you that the biggest fibers are the Mafia hit men of your body. They don't help the underlings collect money from deadbeats. They suit up only when the work calls for their special talents, and when no one else can be trusted to do the job right. In other words, a guy who's trying to build as much muscle as possible must eventually work with weights that require something close to an all-out effort. Otherwise, the highest-threshold fibers would never spring into action. Moreover, the smaller fibers don't need any special high-repetition program of their own, since the size principle also says that if the big fibers are pushed to the max, the small ones are getting blasted, too.

Make sense? Good. Knowing this is the foundation of building the body you want.

YOU CAN IMPROVE MUSCLE QUALITY

On the day you were conceived, the gene gods made three decisions that you might want to quibble with as an adult, if you could:

1. Your maximum number of muscle fibers

2. Your percentages of fast- and slow-twitch fibers

3. The shapes of your muscles when fully developed

On the downside, unless you were born to anchor the 4x100 relay at the next summer Olympics, you can forget about ever reaching that goal. The athletes at the extremes—the fastest and strongest, the ones with the best-looking muscles, and the ones capable of the greatest endurance—were already at the extremes from the moment sperm swam headlong into egg. The upside is that there's a lot of wiggle room in between. Few of us ever approach our full genetic potential. You probably will never be a freak, but with the right kind and amount of work, you can always be a little freakier than you are now. The best way to do that is to learn to use your muscles' very own juice machine.

MORE MUSCLE COMES FROM MORE T

Everyone has some testosterone—babies, little girls playing with tea sets, grandparents shuffling through the laxative aisle at CVS—but no one has hormonal increases from one year to the next like a maturing male. His level increases tenfold during puberty, starting sometime between ages 9 and 15, and he hits near-peak production in his late teens. From there, his testosterone level climbs slowly until about age 30, at which point he hits or passes a few other peaks. His muscle mass will top out between the ages of 18 and 25, unless he intervenes with some barbell therapy. Sexual desire peaks in his early 30s. Sports performance, even among elite athletes, peaks in the late 20s and starts to decline in the early 30s. None of this is inevitable, of course. Unless you're that elite athlete who's trained for his sport since before the short hairs sprouted, you probably have the potential to grow bigger and stronger than you've ever been. And that could also put a little of that teenage explosiveness back into your sex life.

The testosterone/muscle-mass link is pretty clear in general terms: The more you have of one, the more you get of the other. Strength training, while it doesn't necessarily make your testosterone level go up permanently, certainly makes it get a little jiggy in the short term. We know of four ways to create a temporary surge in your most important hormone.

1. Do exercises that employ the most muscle mass, such as squats, deadlifts, pullups, and dips.

2. Use heavy weights, at least 85 percent of the maximum you can lift once on any given exercise.

3. Do a lot of work during your gym time—multiple exercises, multiple sets, multiple repetitions.

4. Keep rest periods fairly short—30 to 60 seconds.

Of course, you can't do all these things in the same workout. For example, when you work a lot of muscle mass with heavy weights, you can't do a high volume of exercise, nor can you work effectively with short rest periods. This is among the many reasons you should periodize your workouts, which is a polysyllabic way of saying change your workouts every few weeks, rather than do the same thing from now till the gene gods recall the merchandise.

Lucky for you, this book is loaded with a variety of workouts that will keep your muscles challenged (almost like we planned it that way, huh?).

MUSCLES NEED MORE THAN PROTEIN

The mythology surrounding protein and muscle building could fill a book, even though the science is fairly straightforward. Your muscles are made of protein (except the four-fifths that's water), so you have to eat protein to make them grow. You also have to eat protein to keep them from shrinking, which is why men trying to lose fat without sacrificing muscle do best when they build their diets around high-quality, muscle-friendly protein from lean meat, fish, eggs, poultry, and low-fat dairy products.

But if you're young, lean, and trying to gain solid weight, a lot of extra protein may not help as much as you think. Protein has qualities that help weight loss and may curtail weight gain. First, protein is metabolically expensive for your body to process. Your body burns about 20 percent of each protein calorie just digesting it. (It burns about 8 percent of carbohydrate and 2 percent of fat during digestion.)

Second, protein creates a high level of satiety, both during meals and between them. In other words, it makes you feel fuller faster and keeps you feeling full longer between meals. (This effect does wear off as you grow accustomed to a higher-protein diet, so it may not have an impact on long-term weight gain or weight loss.)

Finally, if you eat more protein than your body needs, it will learn to use the protein for energy. You want your body to burn carbohydrates and fat for energy, obviously, so a body that's relying on protein for energy is like a car that's using pieces of its engine for fuel.

The best weight-gain strategy is to focus on calories first, protein second. You should make sure you're eating at least 2 grams of protein per kilogram of muscle mass. A kilogram is 2.2 pounds, so a 160-pound guy weighs about 73 kilograms and should take in a minimum of 146 grams protein a day. But that's just 584 calories of protein, the amount you'd find in 15 ounces of chicken, two salmon fillets, or a 28-ounce steak. A protein-powder shake can amp up your totals, as well. If you need to eat more than 3,000 calories a day to gain weight, you'd better have some sweet potatoes with those steaks.

RUN LESS TO GROW FASTER

Running doesn't build muscle mass. If it did, marathoners would have legs like defensive linemen, and workers in Boston would have to repave the streets each year following the city's signature race. But running shrinks muscle fibers to make them more metabolically efficient, thereby saving the pavement.

You'd think you could get around this by lifting weights in addition to running, but your body negates that work through a mysterious "interference effect." Your type II fibers—the biggest ones—will still grow if you run and lift. But your type I fibers won't, and even though they're smaller than the type IIs, they probably comprise 50 percent of the muscle fibers in your body that have any growth potential.

Cut back on your running program and you'll see growth in both your slow- and fast-twitch muscle fibers, and perhaps finally get your body to look the way you think it should.

WHAT IT'S *REALLY* GOING TO TAKE

Fortunately, the body you want (or in most cases, the body you want *back*) can be built (or *re*built). Anyone can shed the fat and rebuild the muscle—or do the opposite, go from scrawny to brawny—if they put in the time and the effort. And that's what it takes—effort. There's no shaping up without sweating and breathing heavy. If anyone tries to tell you otherwise, they are lying. Sure, there are shortcuts—in fact, this book is full of them—but you still have to lift heavy objects regularly, elevate your heart rate and metabolism, and eat fewer Oreos if you want to build a hot body.

Do you want to build a hot body? We thought so. Here's some motivation: By the time you get through the workouts in this book, you can expect to increase the size of your muscle 20 to 40 percent, and not just in your "vanity" muscles, but all over your body. That's what the exercise physiologists tell us is typical of men and women who dedicate themselves to at least a month (and more likely several months) of regular weight training. That's pure bulk. But you'll also enjoy significant gains in strength. Studies show that men can typically boost strength 40 percent.

Think about this every time you pick up a piece of iron: Every time you do a set of resistance exercises, you trigger your body to release chemicals that thicken muscle fibers and help them contract with greater force and efficiency. How? It works like this: Muscles grow through a combination of load and time under tension. By starting each rep with the weights at your sides and then lifting them to your shoulders, for example, you effectively double the amount of time your arm, shoulder, and upper-back muscles spend working.

Let's say you want your construction crew to erect bigger biceps. They'll rely mostly on two key building materials: myofibrils (ropelike strands made up of thinner protein filaments) and sarcoplasm (a gel-like fuel that surrounds the myofibrils). Now, if you lift low reps of heavy weights, the crew will mainly thicken your myofibrils, increasing size and strength. If, on the other hand, you lift high reps of medium weights, those hard hats will primarily boost the volume of your sarcoplasm, building size and endurance.

"Both kinds of growth require stressing your muscles beyond what they're used to, and the way you train dictates which kind of growth you emphasize," says Alexander Koch, Ph.D., C.S.C.S., an associate professor of exercise science at Truman State University.

Here's how each method works your muscles:

When you do a high number of reps with a moderate weight: Some myofibril growth occurs, but your body also sends a signal to increase the size and number of mitochondria, the mini motors inside all your cells.

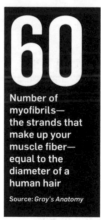

60

Number of myofibrils— the strands that make up your muscle fiber— equal to the diameter of a human hair

Source: *Gray's Anatomy*

As your mitochondria multiply to handle the endurance demands of a high-rep workout, your supply of sarcoplasm also increases to make your muscles function more efficiently. Sarcoplasm is made up of adenosine triphosphate, creatine phosphate, glycogen, and water— a combination that not only transports energy to your muscles but also adds volume to your myofibrils.

When you do a low number of reps with a heavy weight: This causes microtears in your myofibrils. These tears trigger your immune system to send white blood cells to clear away damaged cell fragments, preparing the site for rebuilding. At the same time, your body experiences a boost in human growth hormone, which has a twofold effect: The extra HGH activates dormant stem cells and makes it easier for your body to use the amino acids in protein. Those newly awakened stem cells flock to your injured muscle. There, with the help of the amino acids, they may grow new filaments or fuse with the existing filaments, making your myofibrils denser, larger, and stronger.

WHAT IT ALL MEANS

Put simply: If you hit the workouts in this book, maintaining a variety of exercises and continually challenging your muscles so they, in effect, never get bored, within weeks you'll see your body transform. You'll build muscle, melt away fat, and feel stronger than you ever have.

So . . . what are you waiting for?

All you have to do it read on and get ready to, literally, work your gut off.

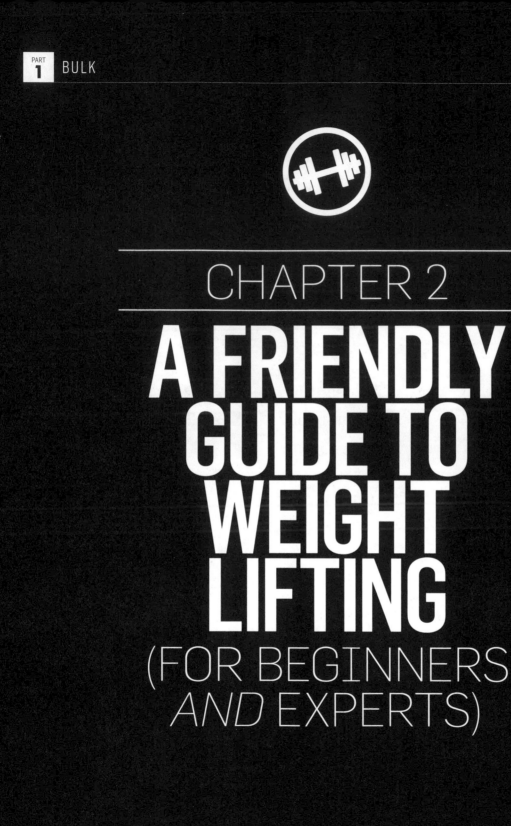

CHAPTER 2

A FRIENDLY GUIDE TO WEIGHT LIFTING

(FOR BEGINNERS *AND* EXPERTS)

W hether you've never lifted a dumbbell or you've spent years in various gyms, it's always good to pay respect to the classics.

Compound exercises like the deadlift, squat, and bench press allow you to handle heavier amounts of weight, for even greater gains in strength—they work more than 85 percent of your body's muscles. Your legs, chest, and back are all primary muscle groups that require other, secondary muscle groups—the shoulders, triceps, biceps, abdominals, and calves—to assist in every exercise. When it comes to a full-body workout, it's crucial to exhaust your primary muscles first and your secondary muscles last. The smartest order: legs first, upper body second, abs last.

The following workout, based on the ultimate heavy-metal classic, the deadlift, is a great way to introduce yourself (or reintroduce, if you've been away) to big-muscle, total-body lifts. The deadlift is a simple, powerful exercise that adds size and strength from head to toe. Done correctly, the move requires many muscles to work together to lift the weight.

HOW TO DO IT

Stand straight with your feet shoulder-width apart and a light barbell on the floor in front of you, with the bar directly over your toes. Bend your knees and grasp the bar with an alternating grip (one palm facing you, the other facing away), your hands just outside your knees. Keeping your head and back straight, slowly stand, keeping the bar close to your body as you lift, until your legs are straight (knees unlocked). Pause, then slowly lower the bar to the floor.

THE PAYOFFS

A better body! Most total-body workouts use compound movements that require many muscles to work together. The end result is greater functional strength that can help improve your athletic performance and daily life.

Bigger muscles! Most compound exercises allow you to lift heavier amounts of weight than other exercises do. The more weight you're able to handle, the more your muscles are forced to grow.

A quicker workout! An exercise plan that targets every major muscle group in one session gives your body a complete workout in less time than a plan that focuses on each muscle group individually.

More power! Explosive movements such as jumping, sprinting, and throwing require all your muscles to work in cooperation. Creating that type of connection is easier when you perform exercises that leave your muscles no choice but to work together.

ARMS. Keep your arms straight throughout the move. Don't shrug your shoulders or bend your elbows to help lift the weight.

ABS. Pull your abs in before you lift. This helps flatten your lower back for better support as you perform the move.

HANDS. Space your hands shoulder-width apart and grab the bar using an alternating grip. Holding the bar this way helps you keep it from slipping.

LEGS. Begin to straighten your legs before you start to pull the weight from the floor so that there's tension in your arms. You should feel the bar comfortably sliding up and down your legs throughout the lift.

HEAD. Keep your head in line with your neck and back at all times. Tilting your head down to look at the bar places stress on your neck and trapezius muscles.

LOWER BACK. Keep your back flat and in line with your head and neck. Arching your back redirects more effort onto your lower-back muscles, placing them at a greater risk of injury.

BUTT. Squeeze your glutes at the start of the movement.

FEET. Your feet should be shoulder-width apart and flat on the floor at all times.

KNEES. Avoid locking your knees as you straighten your legs at the top of the lift.

13

THE WORKOUT

YOUR POWER PLAN

Multijoint exercises can give you the best full-body workout in the shortest time. These five exercises combine compound and functional moves so you'll work as many muscles as possible. After your deadlift routine, pick one exercise from either 1A or 1B (lower body), do the dumbbell bench press (2A, upper body), and pick one move from 3A or 3B (abdominals). Then build your program using the chart below. You'll get a custom-made workout that will improve the strength, size, and performance of every muscle in your body—in less time than you would expect.

THE RIGHT WORKOUT FOR YOU

Build the ultimate physique with our easy-to-use chart.

	BEGINNER	INTERMEDIATE	ADVANCED
WORK YOUR ENTIRE BODY	Three times a week	Twice a week	Twice a week
SETS OF EACH EXERCISE	1–3	2–4	3–5
REPETITIONS PER SET	10–15	8–12	6–8
SPEED OF EACH REPETITION	3–4 seconds up, 3–4 seconds down	2–3 seconds up, 2–3 seconds down	2 seconds up, 2 seconds down
REST BETWEEN SETS	30–60 seconds	60–120 seconds	90–240 seconds

THE EXERCISES

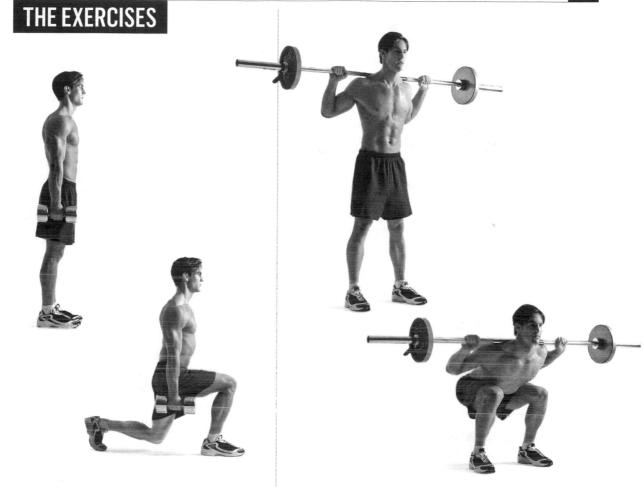

1A. DUMBBELL LUNGE

Stand holding a dumbbell in each hand, arms hanging at your sides, feet about 6 inches apart. Keeping your back straight, step forward with your right foot and lower your body until your right thigh is almost parallel to the floor. Push yourself back up to the starting position and repeat the move, this time stepping out with your left foot.

Get more: Stand with the toes of your right foot resting on a weight bench. Slowly lower yourself into a lunge position. (Your right leg should be used only to help maintain your balance.) Press yourself back up and complete 1 set, then switch legs.

1A. BARBELL SQUAT

Place a barbell on a squat rack at about chest level. Grab the bar with an overhand grip slightly wider than shoulder-width apart, duck underneath it, and rest the bar across the back of your shoulders. Lift the bar off the rack and step back. With your feet shoulder-width apart and your back straight, slowly squat until your thighs are almost parallel to the floor. Pause, then press yourself back up into a standing position.

Get more: Move your left foot forward so it's 2 to 3 feet in front of your right foot. Squat until your left thigh is parallel to the floor, press yourself back up, and complete 1 set before repeating with your right foot in front of your left.

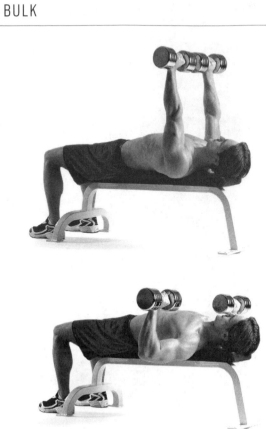

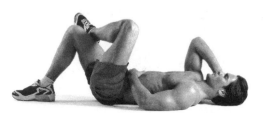

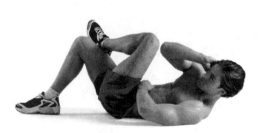

2A. DUMBBELL BENCH PRESS

Grab a dumbbell in each hand (palms forward) and lie on a bench with your feet flat on the floor. Hold your arms straight above your chest. Slowly lower the weights to the sides of your chest. Pause, then press them back up.
Get more: Try doing the move one arm at a time. Start with both weights positioned by the sides of your chest, then slowly press one dumbbell above your chest while keeping the other in place. Lower the weight, then repeat the move with the other weight.

3A. CROSS-KNEE TWISTING CRUNCH

Lie on your back with your knees bent and your feet flat on the floor. Cross your left foot over your right knee. (Your left ankle should rest just below your right knee.) Place your right hand on the back of your head, pointing your elbow forward. (Your left hand can rest on your midsection.) Now, slowly curl your torso off the floor and twist to the left, drawing your right elbow to your left knee. Pause, then lower yourself back down and repeat. Finish the set, then switch leg positions to work the opposite side.
Get more: Straighten your legs and raise them so your feet are about 2 feet above the floor. As you curl your torso, simultaneously bend your knees toward your elbow; as you lower your torso, straighten your legs so your feet return to the starting position.

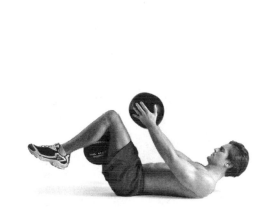

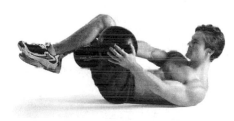

3B. MEDICINE-BALL TWISTING CURL

Lie on your back and place a small medicine ball under your knees. (Draw your feet toward your butt to pinch the ball in place.) Your thighs should be almost perpendicular to the floor. Hold another medicine ball with straight arms pointing at your thighs. Now slowly curl your head and shoulders off the floor and twist to the left. (The ball in your hands should end up at the outside of your left thigh.) Lower yourself, then repeat the move, this time twisting to the right.

Get more: Try holding the ball with your arms extended straight behind your head—your upper arms by your ears—at the start of the move. Then sweep the ball over your head and in front as you curl up and twist.

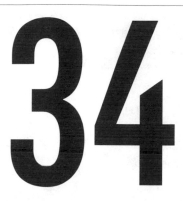

34

Percentage of men who drop pounds by including both weight training and sprinting in their routines

Know Your Muscles

The deadlift involves the erector spinae **(1)**, trapezius **(2)**, latissimus dorsi **(3)**, forearm extensors **(4)**, obliques **(5)**, gluteals **(6)**, and quadriceps **(7)**. Here's how they work together to execute the move.

Challenging Changeup

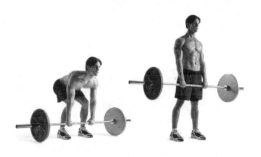

OVERHAND-GRIP DEADLIFT

Get in the same position you use for a regular deadlift, but instead of holding the bar with an alternating grip, grab it with both palms facing you. This traditional hand position is less effective than the alternating grip at maintaining your grip during your heaviest lifts, but it can make the move more comfortable to perform.

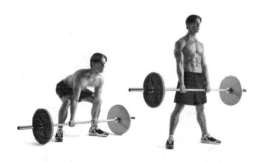

UNDERHAND-GRIP DEADLIFT

Get in the same position you use for a regular deadlift, but instead of holding the bar with an alternating grip, grab it with both palms facing away from you. This traditional hand position is less effective than the alternating grip at maintaining your grip during your heaviest lifts, but it can make the move more comfortable to perform.

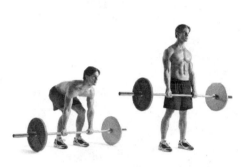

ALTERNATING-GRIP DEADLIFT

At the start of the deadlift, your forearms contract to grip the bar while the latissimus dorsi, trapezius, erector spinae, obliques, and upper and lower rectus abdominis isometrically contract to stabilize your vertebral column. (They stay contracted throughout the lift.) The bar begins to move upward with the initial extension of the gluteal muscles and quadriceps. Your glutes and quads continue to contract as you straighten your legs to pull the weight up along your thighs. At the top of the lift, the trapezius muscles join in to bring your body into a proper upright position. Then, as you lower the bar, your glutes and quads contract to lower the weight while the other muscles stay contracted.

UNILATERAL DUMBBELL DEADLIFT

Place a heavy dumbbell along the outside of your right foot and bend down into the starting position for a deadlift. Grab the weight with your palm facing in, then stand up and lift it, letting your other arm hang at your side. Lifting with only one arm lets you concentrate on one side at a time, while trying to maintain your balance works additional stabilizing muscles in your legs and lower back.

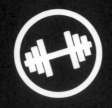

CHAPTER 3

PACK ON 15 POUNDS OF MUSCLE AND GO FROM SCRAWNY TO BRAWNY

If you ask a skinny guy where he wants to grow the most, he'll keep the answer nice and simple: "Chest, shoulders, and biceps, please." Rest assured, this workout can add serious size to those areas. But it'll also muscle up your legs and back. The upshot: You'll look bigger and buffer from every angle.

TARGETS OF OPPORTUNITY

Pectoralis Major

Your main chest muscle is the pectoralis major **(A)**. Its job is to pull your upper arms toward the middle of your body. Think about that in terms of a bench press: As you push the bar away from your torso, your upper arms straighten and move closer to your chest. That's because your pectoralis major attaches to the inside of your upper-arm bone. So when your pectorals contract, the muscle fibers shorten, pulling your upper arms toward the muscles' origin—the middle of your chest. The fibers of your pectoralis major originate at three places on your chest: your collarbone **(B)**, called the clavicular portion, or upper chest; and your breastbone **(C)** and ribs **(D)**, collectively known as the sternal portion, or lower chest.

Front and Middle Deltoids

The roundish-looking muscle that caps the top of your upper arm is called your deltoid. It's the shoulder muscle you show off when you wear a sleeveless shirt. It's made up of three distinct sections: your front deltoid **(E)**, middle deltoid **(F)**, and rear deltoid (not shown). Two of the best exercises for your front and middle delts are bench presses and shoulder presses.

Biceps

When men talk about biceps, they're primarily referring to the biceps brachii **(G).** This muscle starts at your shoulder and attaches to your forearm. Its duties are to bend your elbow and to rotate your forearm. Any type of arm curl works this muscle, as do chinups and rows.

HOW TO PACK ON 15 POUNDS OF MUSCLE

Picture some of college football's biggest, strongest athletes. When it's time for them to go the NFL combine, they train even harder and pack on an extra 10 to 15 pounds of solid muscle. That's right: Some of the best athletes in the country have to jack up their game even higher. What's even more amazing: They do it in a few weeks, using basic exercises. The secret? Maximum effort. They're willing to go all out to achieve what they want. Are you?

DIRECTIONS

Do each workout (A and B) twice a week, with at least one day off before repeating workouts. So if you do A and B on Monday and Tuesday, take Wednesday off. Then repeat A and B on Thursday and Friday. Take an extra day of rest if you're feeling run down or excessively sore. Warm up for 10 minutes. Do the exercises in the order shown. After each set, rest long enough to do the next set with nearly the same level of performance—about 3 minutes for 5-rep sets, and 1½ to 2 minutes for the others. Do one of the core exercises before or after the strength exercises in A and B.

WORKOUT A

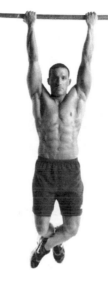

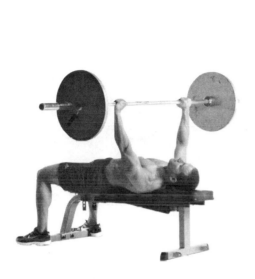

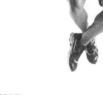

Squeeze your shoulder blades as you pull your chest to the bar.

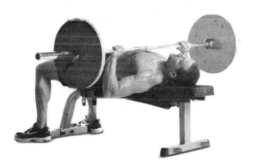

BENCH PRESS

Hold a bar above your chest using an overhand, shoulder-width grip. Lower it to your chest, and press it back up.
Do 3 warmup sets of 5 reps using 75 percent of your estimated max. Then do 4 sets of 5 reps using 85 percent of your max.

CHINUP

Hang at arm's length from a chinup bar using an underhand, shoulder-width grip. This is the starting position. Pull your chest to the bar as fast as you can, pause, and take 2 seconds to lower to the starting position.
Do 4 sets of 6 reps.

WORKOUT A (continued)

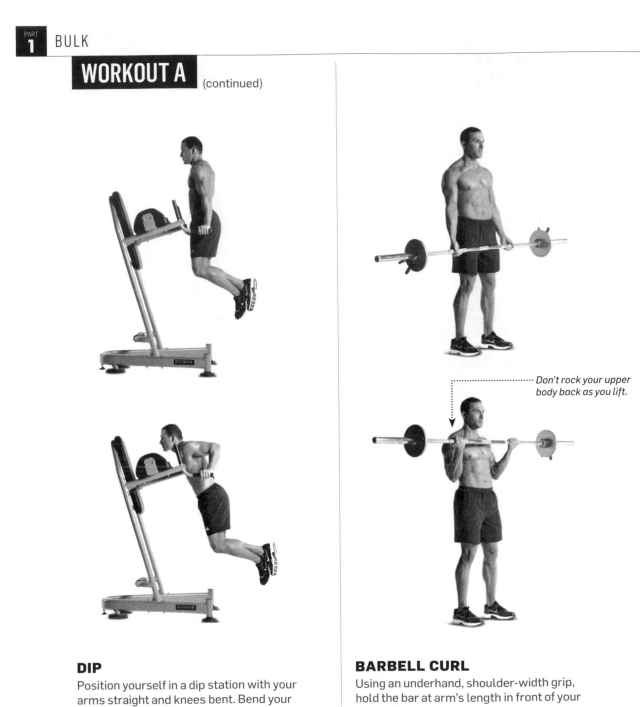

Don't rock your upper body back as you lift.

DIP

Position yourself in a dip station with your arms straight and knees bent. Bend your elbows and lower your body until your elbows are at 90 degrees. Pause for 1 second, and press back up to the starting position.
Do 3 sets of 8 reps.

BARBELL CURL

Using an underhand, shoulder-width grip, hold the bar at arm's length in front of your thighs. Keeping your elbows close to your body, curl the bar up to shoulder level. Pause, lower, and repeat.
Do 3 sets of 8 reps.

WORKOUT B

Keep your torso still at all times.

Don't round your lower back at any time.

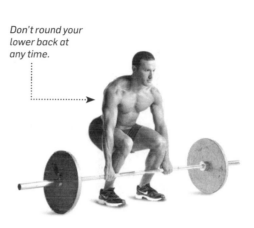

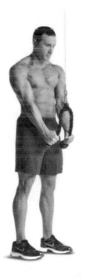

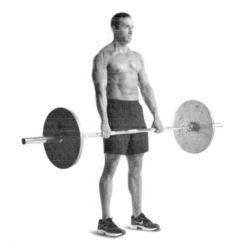

CABLE TRICEPS EXTENSION

Hold the rope attachment of a high pulley of a cable station and stand facing it, your elbows bent 90 degrees. Without moving your upper arms, pull the rope down until your arms are straight. Pause, and repeat.
Do 2 sets of 15 reps.

DEADLIFT

Bend at your hips and knees and grab the bar overhand, your arms just outside your legs. Now stand up, pulling the bar off the floor and thrusting your hips forward.
Do 3 warmup sets of 5 reps using 75 percent of your estimated max. Then do 4 sets of 5 reps using 85 percent of your max.

WORKOUT B (continued)

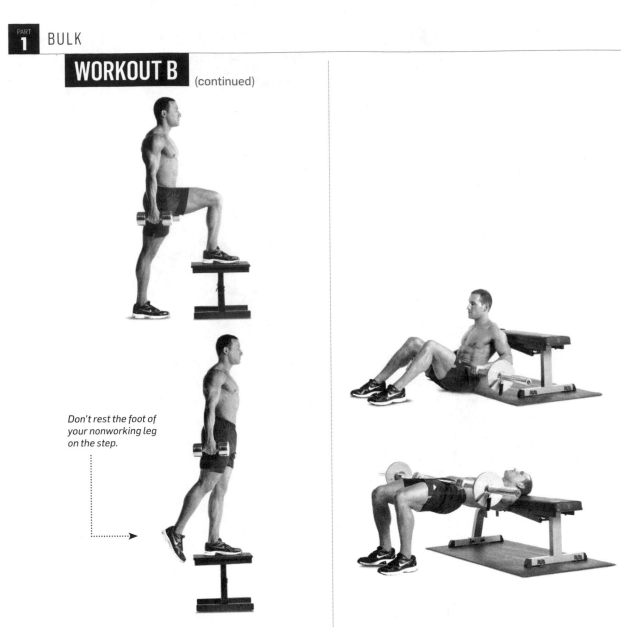

Don't rest the foot of your nonworking leg on the step.

DUMBBELL STEPUP

Grab a pair of dumbbells and place one foot on a bench or step. Press through your heel and lift yourself onto the bench. Take 2 seconds to lower your non-base foot to the floor. Do all your reps, and then switch legs and repeat. **Do 3 sets of 6 reps.**

BARBELL HIP RAISE

Sit on the floor with your shoulder blades against a bench, your knees bent, and your feet flat. Place a bar across your hips; this is the starting position. Squeezing your glutes, lift your hips until your body forms a straight line from your shoulders to your knees. Lower, and repeat. **Do 3 sets of 8 reps.**

CORE WORKOUT

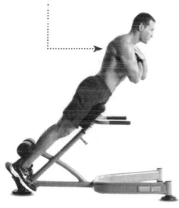

To make it harder, hold a weight across your chest.

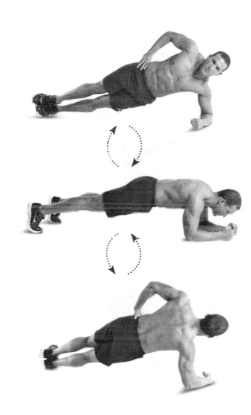

BACK EXTENSION

Hook your heels into a back extension station. Keeping your back naturally arched, lower your torso until your body is bent 90 degrees. Then raise your torso back up until it's in line with your lower body. Hold this position for 3 seconds.
Do 3 sets of 8 reps.

BEGINNER
ROLLING PLANK

Start in a pushup position but with your weight on your forearms. Brace your core and hold for 30 seconds. Now roll to your left into a side plank and hold for 30 seconds. Then roll to the original plank position and hold for 30 seconds. Roll to your right for a 30-second side plank and then return to the original plank and hold for 30 more. That's 1 set.
Do 2 sets, with 1 to 2 minutes of rest between sets.

CORE WORKOUT (continued)

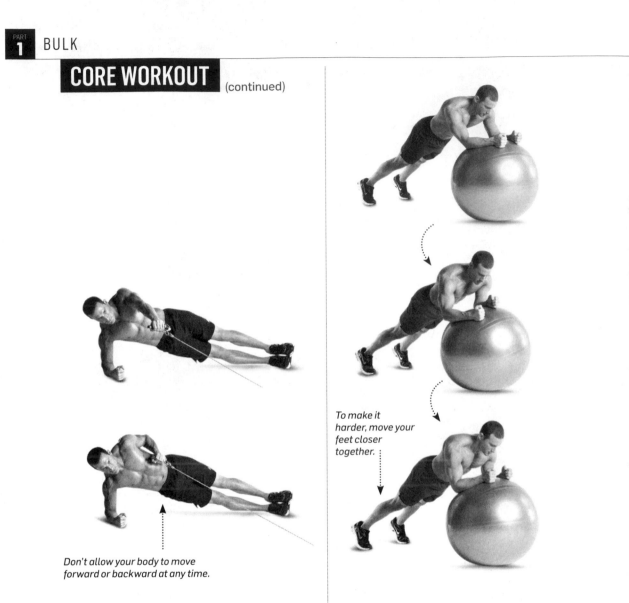

To make it harder, move your feet closer together.

Don't allow your body to move forward or backward at any time.

MODERATE
SIDE PLANK AND ROW

Attach a handle to the low pulley of a cable station and lie on your right side, facing the stack. Grab the handle with your left hand and assume a side plank. Hold the side plank as you pull the handle to your rib cage, pause, and extend your arm. That's 1 rep. Do all your right-side reps, and switch sides and repeat. **Do 3 sets of 10 reps, with 1 minute of rest between sets.**

HARD
SWISS-BALL "STIR THE POT"

Assume a plank position with your forearms on a Swiss ball. Use your forearms to move the ball in small circles while keeping the rest of your body in the original position. Make 10 circles to the left and then 10 to the right. That's 1 set. **Do 3 sets, with 30 seconds of rest between sets.**

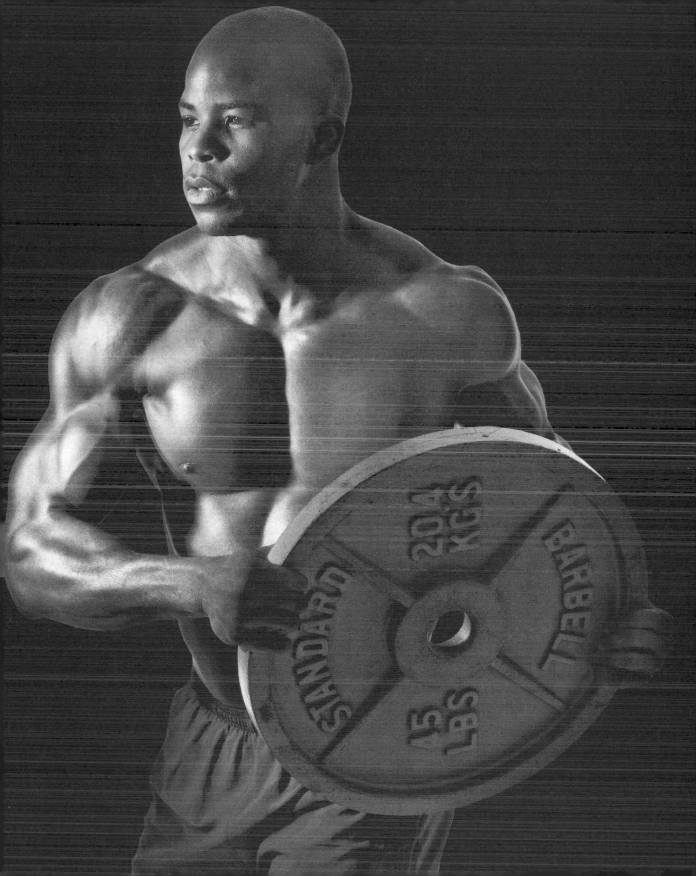

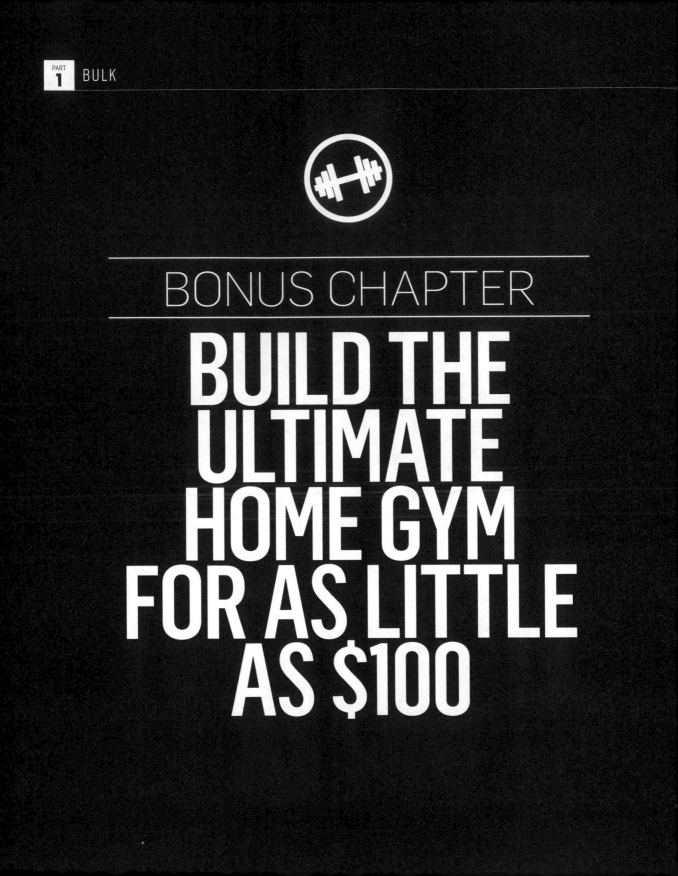

BONUS CHAPTER

BUILD THE ULTIMATE HOME GYM FOR AS LITTLE AS $100

W

orking out at home has a lot of benefits:

- 24/7 access to "the gym"
- No wasted travel time
- No waiting for the bench press
- Really cheap monthly membership fee: $0
- Reduced risk of athlete's foot infections
- Better music: your own
- No glowering dudes wearing cut-off Slayer concert Ts
- Chinup bar doubles as clothes hanger

And when your workout facility is 10 steps from your bedroom, it's harder to find an excuse not to exercise. Of course, there is one downside to working out at home rather than at a gym or health club: You need to buy some gear.

Body-weight exercises are terrific, but they can take you only so far. They "can help you stay lean," says Alwyn Cosgrove, C.S.C.S., co-owner of Results Fitness in Santa Clarita, California. "But to add muscle and torch fat faster, you need tools that add to the difficulty of those movements, and you need some iron."

Fortunately, muscular arms and legs don't have to cost an arm and a leg. You can bulk up no matter what your bankroll. Let's take a look at some options for the do-it-yourselfer.

$100 OR LESS

A stability ball (around $23) **(A)**, also called a Swiss ball. The instability of a Swiss ball increases the challenge of almost every kind of exercise. Use the 65-centimeter (diameter) ball if you're shorter than 6 feet, and a 75-centimeter ball if you're taller.

A pair of dumbbells (around $70). Dumbbells are the ultimate workout tools. Buy them used and you should be able to get two pair for that price, one lightweight and one heavy.

$300 OR LESS

Stability ball, dumbbells, and . . .

Adjustable Weight Bench ($200). A bench is essential for the pressing exercises that help you sculpt a powerful chest and bigger shoulders and arms.

$500 OR LESS

Stability ball, three pairs of dumbbells, adjustable bench, and . . .

Perfect Pullup ($100) **(B)**. Unlike most pullup bars, this version has adjustable handles, which allow you to perform a variety of chinups and pullups, as well as inverted rows. The benefit: more muscle on your back, shoulders, and arms.

Or . . .

TRX Suspension Trainer ($150) **(C)**. This system of nylon straps anchors to something sturdy, such as a door frame, so you can work your legs, core, and upper body.

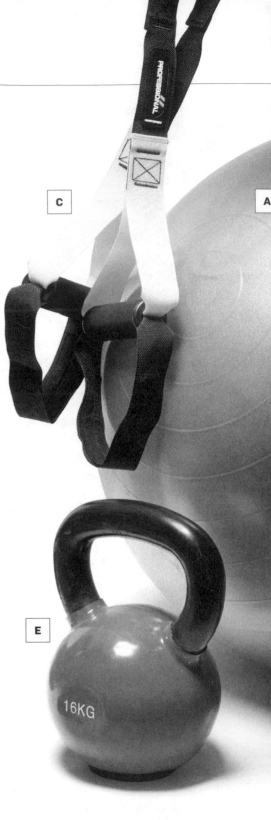

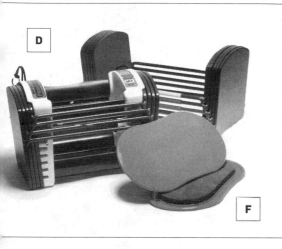

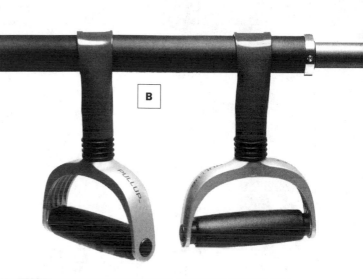

$1,000 OR LESS

Stability ball, four pairs of dumbbells, adjustable bench, pullup bar or suspension trainer, and . . .

300-pound Olympic Barbell Set with Bar, Plates, and Collars (about $500).

As you gradually build your stash of gear, you might also consider:

PowerBlocks ($300) (D)

This 50-pound set of adjustable dumbbells can replace the 22 pairs of traditional dumbbells your gym stocks. Plus, they fit in your closet.

Kettlebell ($80) (E)

Basically, these are cannonballs with handles. They are best for a workout that combines cardio and strength training, adding a twist to such conventional moves as squats, shoulder presses, and curls. They are especially useful for compound moves, such as kettlebell swings that work multiple muscle groups.

The CoreSlider ($25) (F)

Using slides for body-weight exercises (like pushups, lunges, or planks) increases the number of muscles you recruit. The result: bigger strength gains.

Exercise Bands and Resistance Tubing ($10 to $40)

Great to pack for travel, these lightweight tools allow you to do dozens of resistance exercises in a wide range of motion.

Medicine Balls with Handles ($30 to $100)

These weighted rubber balls with one or two integrated handles allow you to easily add weight to body-weight exercises like lunges, rotations, and chops. Smart Bells are another option. The curved, oval platter-sized plates with a handle cut out of each side can be used for doing regular and oblique crunches while holding the weight behind your head, or doing circles, in which you extend the weight above your head with both hands and move your arms in a circular motion in front of your body.

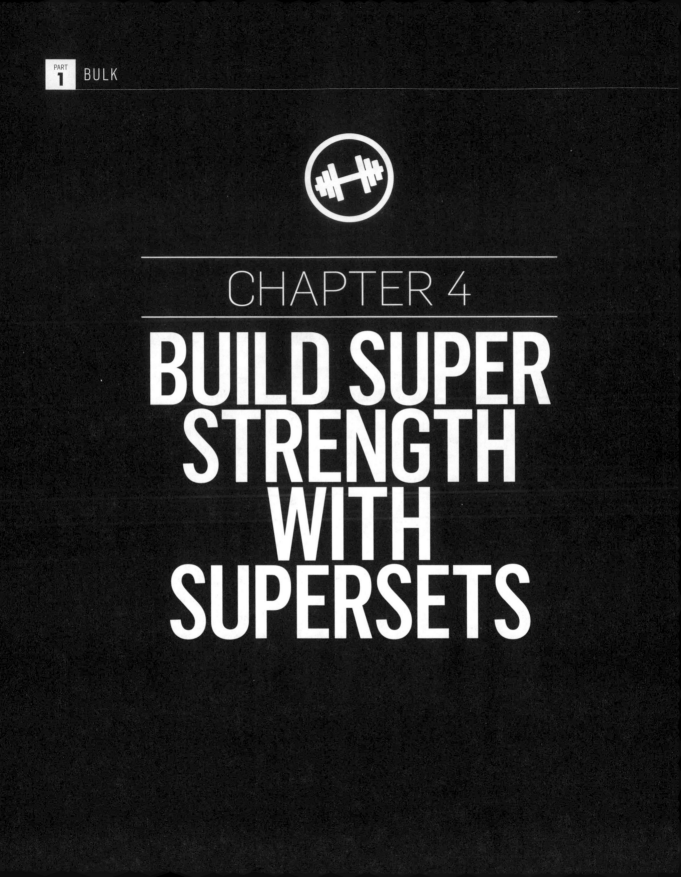

CHAPTER 4

BUILD SUPER STRENGTH WITH SUPERSETS

You've been told to listen to your body, learn its idiosyncrasies, embrace it like a friend. Don't buy it. You can listen and learn, sure, but forget the friendly stuff. When it comes to muscle, you need to be less good buddy and more psychotic drill sergeant. Keep your muscles off balance. When they get used to lifting a certain amount in a certain way (sound like your workout?), they stop growing. A training program that never changes also creates strength imbalances; that's unproductive and dangerous.

This doesn't mean you have to master the incline behind-the-back modified Slovenian triceps windmill. Just do your usual exercises, but use different combinations of sets and repetitions.

What follows is a guide to different kinds of sets and how they produce different results, from trainer Craig Ballantyne, M.S., C.S.C.S., owner of WorkoutManuals.com. Plug this into your gym routine and see the surprised—and supersized—reaction you get from your muscles.

STRAIGHT SETS

What they are: The usual—a number of repetitions followed by a rest period, then by 1 or more sets of the same exercise.

Why they're useful: The rest periods and narrow focus of straight sets help add mass and build maximal strength. As long as you rest enough between sets (1 to 3 minutes), your muscle, or group of muscles, will work hard two, three, even five times in a workout.

How to use them: The start of your workout is the best time to do straight sets, regardless of your experience level, Ballantyne says. Your energy and focus are high at the start, so it's the best time to execute difficult moves. Perform 3 straight sets of 6 to 8 repetitions of a challenging exercise like the bench press, pullup, or squat; aim to do the same number of repetitions in each set, with either the same or increasing amounts of weight.

SUPERSETS

What they are: A set of each of two different exercises performed back-to-back, without rest.

Why they're useful: Supersets save time and burn fat. You can multitask your muscles—for instance, working your chest and back in one superset and legs and shoulders in another. Lifting heavy weights in a short time period increases the rate at which your body breaks down and rebuilds protein. This metabolism boost lasts for hours after you've finished lifting.

How to use them: Insert a superset at any time in your workout. To involve the most muscles, pair compound exercises—moves that work multiple muscles across multiple joints. For example, combine a chest press with a row, or a shoulder press with a deadlift. To save more time, pair noncompeting muscle groups, such as your deltoids and glutes. One muscle group is able to recover while the other works, so you can repeat the set without resting as long.

TRISETS

What they are: Three different exercises performed one after another, without any rest in between.

Why they're useful: Trisets save time and raise metabolism. A single triset can be a total-body workout in itself, like a *Men's Health* 15-Minute Workout.

33

Percentage more calories you burn after doing supersets (back-to-back sets of two different exercises) compared with sets that let you rest between moves

Source: *The Journal of Strength and Conditioning Research*

How to use them: Trisets are a good workout for at home (or in an empty gym), because you need to monopolize equipment for three exercises. Do basic exercises that hit different body parts—like bench presses, squats, and chinups. Perform a warmup set using 50 percent of the weight you usually use in each exercise. Then repeat the triset two or three times, using weights that allow you to perform 8 repetitions per set. Rest 1 to 3 minutes after each triset.

DROP SETS

What they are: Three or 4 sets of one exercise performed without rest, using a lighter weight for each successive set. Also called descending sets or strip sets.

Why they're useful: Drop sets are a great quick workout, fatiguing your muscles in a short time, getting your heart going, and giving you an impressive postworkout pump as your muscles fill with blood.

How to use them: Use drop sets when you're pressed for time. Don't do them more than three times a week; you'll get so tired you won't be able to accomplish much else. Start with a warmup, using 50 percent of the weight you expect to use in your first set. Now use the heaviest weight you'd use for 8 repetitions of that exercise to perform as many repetitions as you can. Drop 10 to 20 percent of the weight and go again. Continue to reduce the weight and go again, always trying to complete the same number of repetitions (even though you won't), until your muscles fail.

CIRCUIT SETS

What they are: A series of exercises (usually six) that you complete one after another without rest, though you can do some cardiovascular work (such as jumping rope) between exercises.

Why they're useful: When you use weights, circuits can be a great total-body workout. But they're most valuable without weights as a warmup of the nervous system, joints, and muscles, Ballantyne says. Because a circuit stresses the entire body, it's more effective than a treadmill jog, which primes only your lower body.

How to use them: You'll annoy the other guys at the gym if you do an entire workout based on circuits, because you'll monopolize so many pieces of equipment. But one circuit is quick and effective. If you're using it as a warmup, you need only your body weight or a barbell. Or use just a pair of dumbbells and circuit-train at home where you won't annoy anyone.

THE COMBO-PLATTER WORKOUT

This full-body workout from Craig Ballantyne, C.S.C.S., runs the gamut of sets. It focuses on two often-neglected areas: the upper back and the "posterior chain"—the hamstrings, glutes, and lower back. The posterior chain gives you power and speed in sports.

WARMUP CIRCUIT

This is an all-purpose warmup for any strength-training workout.
All you need is a barbell. Do 8 repetitions of each exercise and repeat the circuit twice.
- Squat (body weight only)
- Pushup (body weight only)
- Reverse Lunge (body weight only)
- Barbell Row (bar only)
- Diagonal Lunge (body weight only)

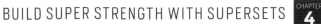
STRAIGHT SETS

SUPERSET #1

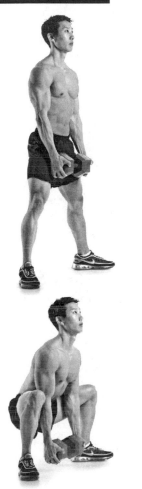

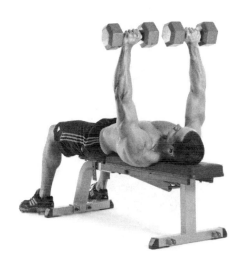

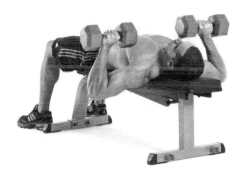

SUMO SQUAT

Stand with your feet more than shoulder-width apart, toes slightly turned out. Hold a dumb-bell between your legs with both hands under the top of the dumbbell. Keep your arms against your body. Squat down until the dumbbell touches the floor, pause, then return to the starting position.
Perform 3 sets of 6 repetitions.
Rest for 2 to 3 minutes after each set.

DUMBBELL CHEST PRESS

Lie on a bench, holding a pair of dumbbells directly over your chest with straight arms and an overhand grip (palms facing away from you). Keep your feet flat on the floor and angled to the sides for better balance. Next, bend your arms to lower the dumbbells to the outsides of your chest, pause, then push the weights back up to the starting position.
Do 8 repetitions of each exercise without resting between the two exercises. Complete 3 supersets, resting for 1 minute after each.

SUPERSET #2

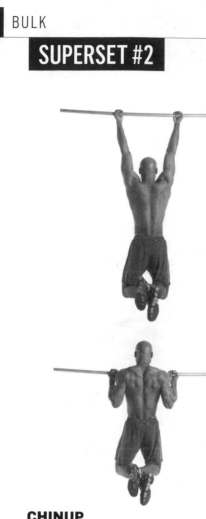

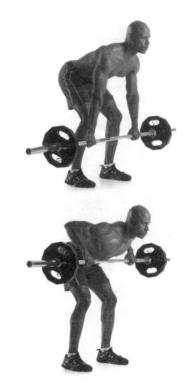

CHINUP

Grab a chinup bar with an underhand grip—
that is, with your palms facing you. Your hands
should be slightly more than shoulder-width
apart. Keeping your head, shoulders, hips,
and knees perfectly aligned, pull your chest
to the bar, pause for a second, and then lower
yourself until your arms are straight again.
Resist locking your elbows, to keep the
tension on your back.
**Do 12 repetitions of each move with no
rest. Rest 1 minute before repeating the
superset. Complete 3 supersets.**

BARBELL ROW

Hold a barbell with an overhand grip and
stand with your knees slightly bent. Bend at
the hips until your torso is almost parallel to
the floor. Your arms should hang straight
down. Pull the bar up until it's even with your
lower rib cage. Pause, then lower the bar
to the starting position.

DROP SETS

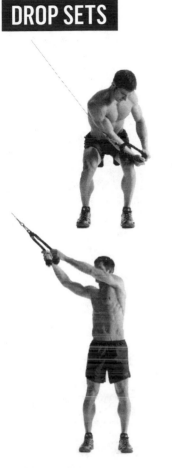

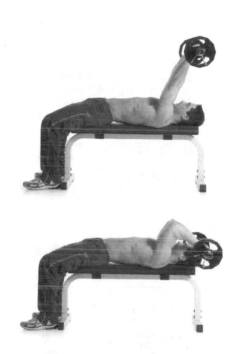

CABLE LIFT

Attach a stirrup handle to a low-pulley cable and stand with your right foot next to the weight stack. Bend your knees and push your hips back to lower yourself into a squat. Reach across your body with straight arms and grab the handle. Keeping your abs tight and elbows locked, stand up and rotate your torso, bringing the handle above your opposite shoulder. Then slowly return to the squat position. After 6 repetitions, turn around and repeat the move with your left foot next to the stack.
Do 4 sets of as many repetitions as possible, beginning with the most weight you can lift eight times and removing 10 to 20 percent of the weight after each set.

LYING TRICEPS EXTENSION

Lie on a bench, holding an EZ-curl bar with an overhand, shoulder-width grip. Hold the bar at arm's length over your forehead. Keeping your upper arms in the same position throughout the move, bend at the elbows to lower the bar to the top of your forehead. Pause, then push the weight back up.

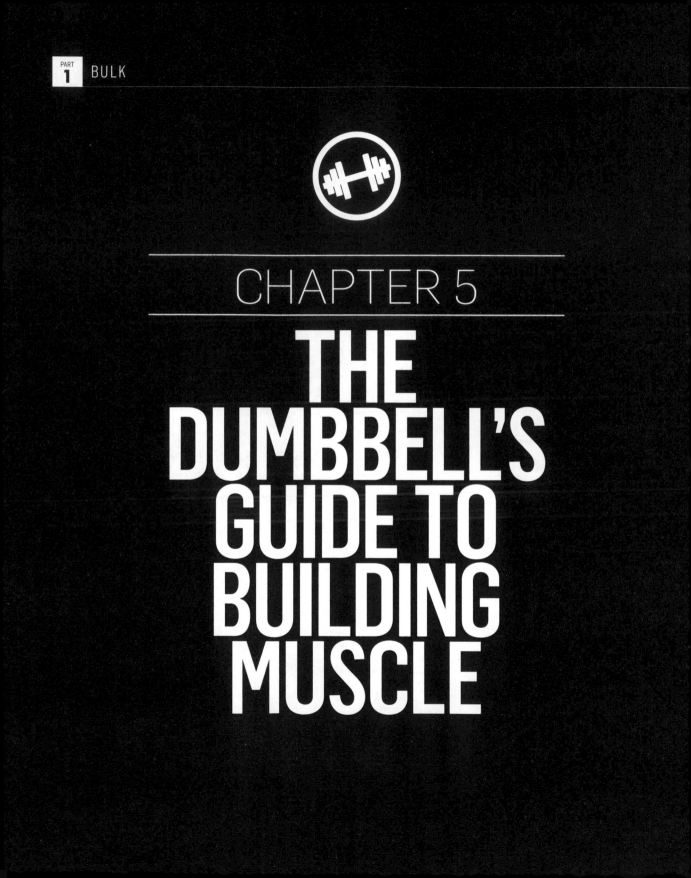

CHAPTER 5

THE DUMBBELL'S GUIDE TO BUILDING MUSCLE

THE TYPICAL HEALTH CLUB WEIGHT ROOM is a lot like an all-you-can eat buffet on the Vegas strip. Rows upon rows of glistening machines are as necessary for a good workout as 150 items are to a belly-filling lunch. You just don't need all that extra stuff—nor the floor-to-ceiling mirrors, track lighting, and antibacterial gel dispensers.

If you asked most strength coaches to choose between training in one of those fancy fitness studios or a concrete-floored room with a couple of cinder blocks and a pipe, most would probably choose the latter. And not because they're old-school or allergic to Purell.

Basic free weights simply test your muscles in ways many machines can't.

The gleaming-chrome machines look high-tech and advanced, but they are actually quite limiting. Most allow you to perform what's called single-joint exercises, where your range of motion is limited to one plane. Leg extensions, biceps curls, and bench presses are good examples when done on machines. Because the machine is designed to lock you into moving in only one direction every time, only a small targeted section of muscle actually receives the bulk of the resistance work. That's better than nothing, but if you really want to build muscle mass and gain strength, training with free weights helps you develop your synergistic muscles—the wide range of muscles that support the bones of the muscles that you are trying to strengthen. Unlike resistance machines, free weights require you to balance the weight, which calls upon many more stabilizing muscles and makes the exercise that much more difficult, requiring greater exertion, which in turn burns more calories. And no free weight is better at that—or more versatile as a strength-building tool—than the simple dumbbell. Just learning how to bench press a pair of unwieldy dumbbells in a biomechanically efficient pattern takes skill, forces your muscles to adapt, and results in increased force production.

So buy yourself some dumbbells and save hundreds of dollars on a health-club membership and your precious time. Crowded gyms can slow your workout—and your results. After all, every second you spend waiting for the chinup bar, cable station, or squat rack is less time you have for working your muscles or igniting your metabolism. More time waiting means less intensity and dramatically reduces your chances of achieving fast, quantifiable results.

Men's Health fitness expert Craig Ballantyne, M.S., C.S.C.S., designed this fat-burning, muscle-building workout, which requires minimal equipment and a small space to exercise. In fact, all you need are a single set of dumbbells and an adjustable bench. The order in which you perform the exercises—along with the number of repetitions for each—allows the same pair of dumbbells to challenge each muscle equally. Without a doubt, this is one of the simplest yet most effective workouts for chiseling a better body.

THE DETAILS

This 3-day-a-week total-body program contains three different dumbbell workouts: A, B, and C. Perform each once a week, resting at least a day between sessions. Within each workout, alternate sets between exercises of the same number (1A and 1B, for example) until you complete all sets in that pairing. (In other words, follow a set of the first exercise with a set of the second exercise.) Rest 1 minute between 1A and 1B, but perform exercises 2A and 2B back-to-back, with no rest. (This adds a nice metabolic circuit effect to the workout.)

After you've done a set of each exercise pair, rest for 1 minute and then repeat the cycle until you've completed all the sets. Then move to the second pair of exercises. Take care to use perfect form. Cheating by using momentum to help you lift the weight only compromises your progress.

Here's a sample workout schedule. You can start workout A on any day of the week. Just be sure to leave at least a day in between workouts to rest and recover.

MONDAY

WORKOUT A

1A. Dumbbell Chest Press
3 sets of 8 reps

1B. Dumbbell Bent-Over Row
3 sets of 12 reps

2A. Dumbbell Squat
2 sets of 5 reps; no rest between the 2A–2B pair

2B. Dumbbell Incline Press
2 sets of 15 reps

TUESDAY

Rest

WEDNESDAY

WORKOUT B

1A. Dumbbell Split Squat
3 sets of 8 reps

1B. Single-Arm Standing Shoulder Press
3 sets of 12 reps

2A. Dumbbell Romanian Deadlift
2 sets of 10 reps; no rest between the 2A–2B pair

2B. Dumbbell Swings
2 sets of 20 reps

THURSDAY

Rest

FRIDAY

WORKOUT C

1A. Dumbbell Stepup
3 sets of 8 reps

1B. Chest-Supported Incline Row
3 sets of 12 reps

2A. Dumbbell Curl
2 sets of 10 reps; no rest between the 2A–2B pair

2B. Lying Dumbbell Triceps Extension
2 sets of 12 reps

SATURDAY

Optional cross-training

SUNDAY

Rest

WORKOUT A

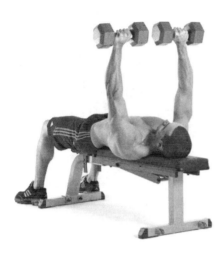

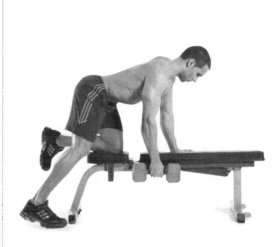

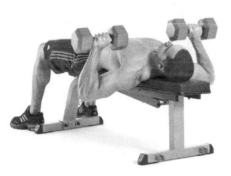

1A. DUMBBELL CHEST PRESS

Lie on your back on a flat bench and hold a pair of dumbbells above your chest with your arms straight. Lower the dumbbells to the sides of your chest, pause, and then push them back up to the starting position.
Do 3 sets of 8 reps.

1B. DUMBBELL BENT-OVER ROW

With a dumbbell in your right hand, place your left hand and left knee on a flat bench. Keep your back flat and let your right arm hang straight down with your palm facing in. Pull your arm up to the side of your chest by bending your elbow. Pause, and return to the starting position.
Do 3 sets of 12 reps for each arm.

WORKOUT A (continued)

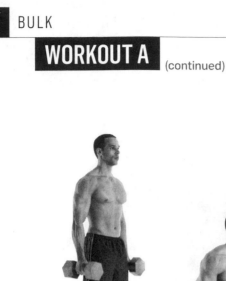

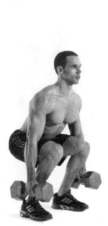

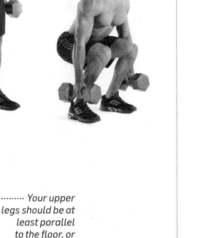

Your upper legs should be at least parallel to the floor, or even lower.

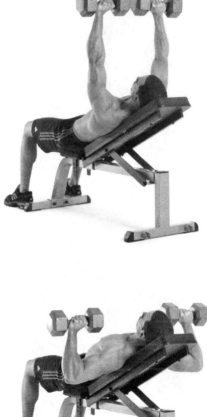

2A. DUMBBELL SQUAT

Holding a pair of dumbbells at your sides, stand with your feet just beyond shoulder-width apart. Push your hips back and squat as deeply as possible, keeping your lower back naturally arched. Push back up to the starting position without rounding your back.
Do 2 sets of 5 reps; no rest between the 2A–2B pair.

2B. DUMBBELL INCLINE PRESS

Lie on a bench with the backrest set at a 45-degree incline. Hold a pair of dumbbells above your chest with palms facing your feet. Lower the weights to chest level, and then press them back to the starting position.
Do 2 sets of 15 reps.

WORKOUT B

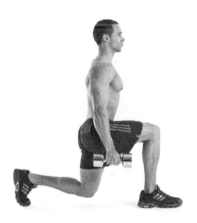

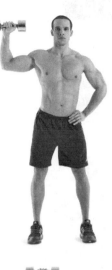

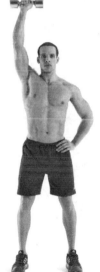

1A. DUMBBELL SPLIT SQUAT

Hold dumbbells at your sides and stand with your right foot forward and your left foot back. Lower your body until your front knee is bent 90 degrees and your rear knee nearly touches the floor. Return to the starting position. Do 8 reps, switch legs, and repeat.

That's 1 set. Do 3 sets of 8 reps.

1B. SINGLE-ARM STANDING SHOULDER PRESS

Stand holding a dumbbell at eye level, with your arm bent, palm forward. Press the dumbbell straight overhead, and then lower it to the starting position. Do 12 reps on one side and repeat with your other arm.

That's 1 set. Do 3 sets of 12 reps.

WORKOUT B (continued)

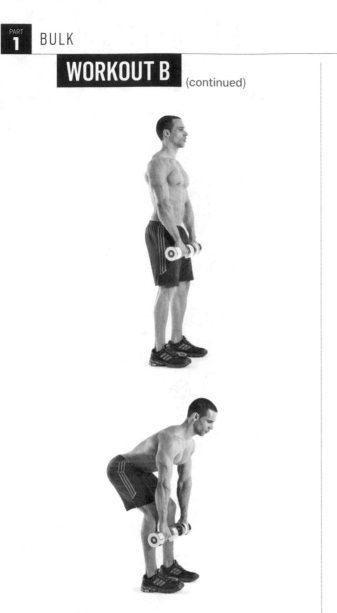

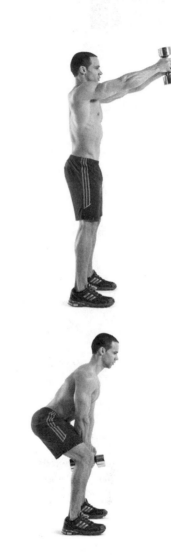

2A. DUMBBELL ROMANIAN DEADLIFT

Hold a dumbbell in each hand in front of your thighs, palms facing your body. With your knees slightly bent and your feet shoulder-width apart, bend at your hips and lower your torso until it's nearly parallel to the floor. Pause, and then rise to the starting position. **Do 2 sets of 10 reps; no rest between the 2A–2B pair.**

2B. DUMBBELL SWINGS

With your feet shoulder-width apart, hold a dumbbell's handle with both hands. Extend your arms in front of your chest. Next, slightly bend your knees and swing the dumbbell between your legs. Bring the dumbbell back up to chest level as you rise. That's 1 rep. **Do 2 sets of 20 reps.**

WORKOUT C

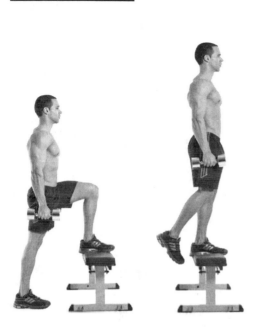

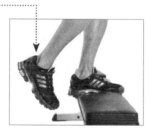

Avoid touching the bench, to keep all the tension on your working leg.

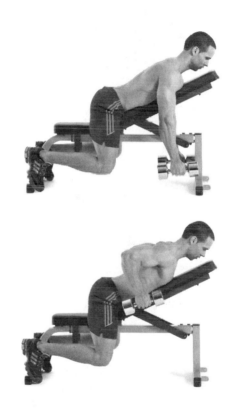

1A. DUMBBELL STEPUP

With a dumbbell in each hand, stand facing a bench and place one foot on the bench. Lift your body up to the standing position without letting your opposite foot touch the bench. Lower your body slowly and repeat. Complete 8 reps, switch legs, and repeat. That's 1 set. **Do 3 sets of 8 reps.**

1B. CHEST-SUPPORTED INCLINE ROW

Grab a pair of dumbbells and lie chest-down on a 45-degree incline bench. Let your arms hang straight down, palms facing each other. Row the dumbbells to the sides of your chest by bending your elbows and squeezing your shoulder blades. Pause, and lower the weights. **Do 3 sets of 12 reps.**

WORKOUT C (continued)

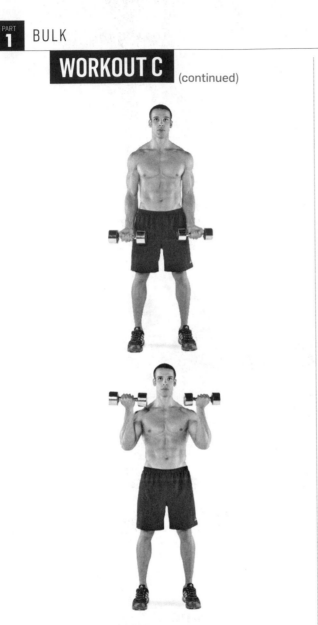

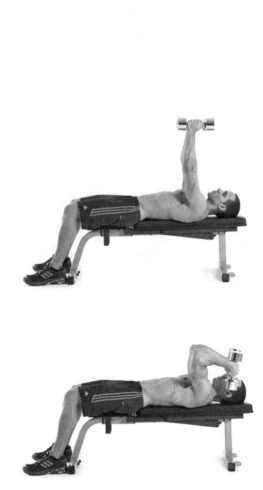

2A. DUMBBELL CURL

Grab a pair of dumbbells with an underhand grip and hold them at arm's length next to your thighs. Curl the dumbbells toward your chest as far as you can without moving your upper arms. Pause and slowly lower the weights to the starting position.
Do 2 sets of 10 reps; no rest between the 2A–2B pair.

2B. LYING DUMBBELL TRICEPS EXTENSION

Hold dumbbells above your chest, palms facing in. Keeping your upper arms still, bend your elbows and move the weights toward your ears. Straighten your arms and repeat.
Do 2 sets of 12 reps.

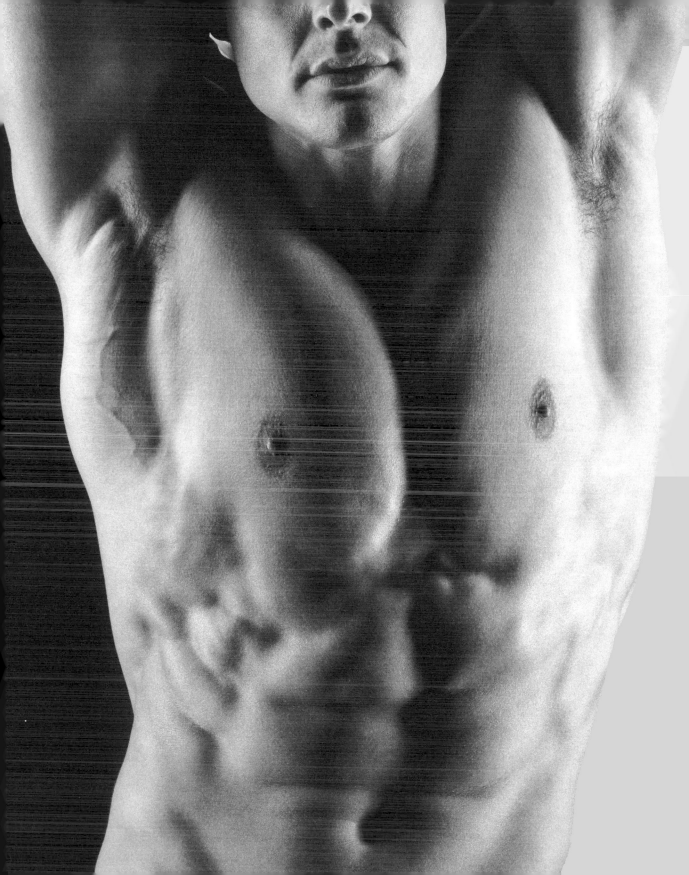

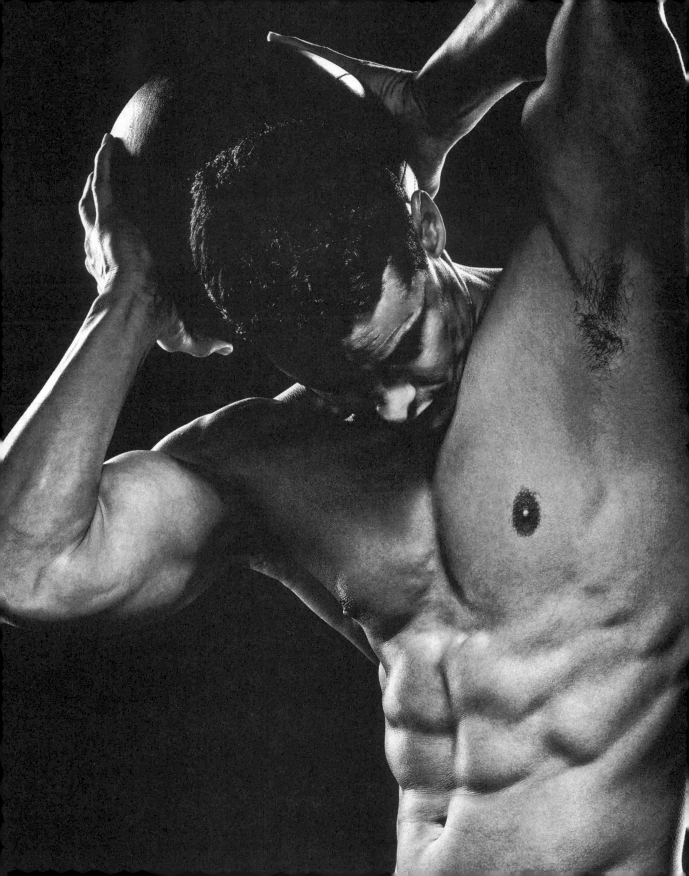

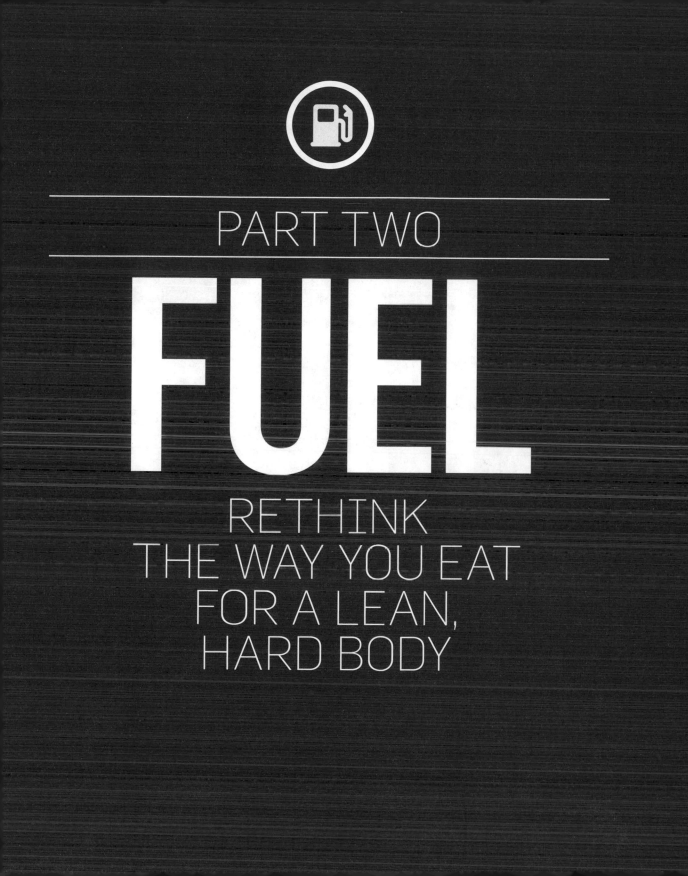

PART TWO

FUEL

RETHINK
THE WAY YOU EAT
FOR A LEAN,
HARD BODY

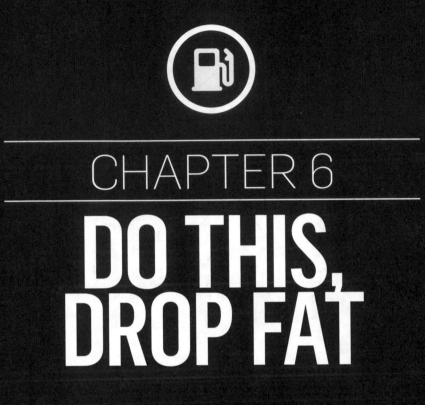

CHAPTER 6

DO THIS, DROP FAT

Your goal: Lose 10 or more pounds of hideous fat.

Why is that so darn hard to do? Because most of us are simply not realistic (and truthful to ourselves) about how much we eat and how little we exercise. Typically, we underestimate the former and overestimate the latter. And we tend to completely banish from our brains all memory of that fourth slice of pizza, the fifth beer, the handful of Hershey's Kisses we scarfed down at mom's house because they were right there in a bowl in front of our noses sweetly calling to us . . . EAT MEEEEEEEEEE!

Yes, we do. Even you.

A fat belly doesn't appear one day like a big zit. It grows gradually, the result of many months and years of flab habits. You know you've got 'em. Time to fess up, because even the most frozen-solid bad eating habits can be broken. It's a matter of identifying them and slowly, deliberately working to change your behavior. And remember this: The less body fat you carry, the quicker your abs will show and develop that Greek-godlike ripple you've always dreamed of. Remember this, too. By breaking some well-entrenched flab habits, you automatically and significantly improve your health. The upsides of a little behavioral modification are enormous.

Start by doing an analysis of your eating habits and then performing triage. A lot easier than it sounds; you'll see. Begin with a pen and a piece of paper. Keeping a food diary is one of the easiest and most efficient ways to get a picture of what, when, and how much you're eating. (See, we even give you sheets of paper to do this self-assessment on page 65: "Action Plan: Keep a Food Journal." All you need is a writing utensil.) In just 3 to 5 days' time, a fascinating snapshot of your flab habits will emerge right before your eyes: your secret Oreo obsession; your tendency to eat three servings at dinnertime; an honest count of bottles of beer you consumed. It'll be an eye-opener. Guaranteed.

Next, target one or two of those behaviors that you feel would give you the most bang for your buck. Take a moment to think about your typical day, and pick your worst habit. Then work for a week on eliminating that habit. Can't accomplish it? Then give yourself another week, until you've wrestled away the habit's grip on your life. The following week, move to your next-weakest link. Focus all your effort on that flab habit while maintaining military-school discipline on your recently banished first flab habit. The key is to take baby steps, not to be overly ambitious in turning your diet around in one fell swoop. We have only so much willpower, a study in *Psychology and Health* shows. That's why trying to break more bad habits at once can be overwhelming: "You drain your capacity for willpower—what researchers call self-regulation," says study author Kathleen Martin Ginis, Ph.D., a professor of kinesi-

Extra-Value Deal
BUILD A BETTER BAKED POTATO
Scoop out the flesh of a baked potato and mash it with steamed broccoli and cottage cheese to add protein and calcium. Stuff the filling back into the skin.

ology at McMaster University in Ontario. This is one time when being too aggressive can backfire.

In this chapter, we'll explore ten of the most common bad eating habits. Chances are excellent that at least a few of these will be revealed through your own food journal. Each flab habit description comes with practical tips and attitude adjustments to help you achieve your weight-loss goals. It won't be long before you notice that your gut is shrinking, your pants are looser, and your abs are breaking out of hiding.

FLAB HABIT #1
SKIPPING MEALS OR SNACKS
Not eating enough (or at all) can mess with your body's ability to control your appetite. But it also destroys willpower, which is just as damaging. "Regulating yourself is a brain activity, and your brain runs on glucose," explains Martin Ginis. If you skip breakfast, lunch, or a healthy snack, then your brain doesn't have enough energy to say no to the inevitable chowfest that occurs later in the day. Skipping a feeding helps turn us into gluttons at night. Your starving brain "just doesn't have the fuel it needs to keep you on track, monitoring your diet."

The worst meal to skip, of course, is breakfast, and not just because grandma said so. Think about it: Since you've been sleeping (and not eating) from 11 p.m. until 6 a.m., if you skip breakfast and eat nothing until lunchtime, you prolong that fast for up to 13 hours. Not eating for 13 hours may sound like an achievement worthy of an attaboy. But it's not. It's stupid. A University of Massachusetts study showed that men who skip their morning meal are 4½ times more likely to have bulging bellies than those who don't. So within an hour of waking, have a meal or protein shake with at least 250 calories. The science: British researchers found that breakfast size was inversely related to waist size. That is, the larger the morning meal, the leaner the midsection. But keep the meal's size within reason: A 1,480 calorie smoked-sausage scramble at the local diner is really two breakfasts, so cap your intake at 500 calories. For a quick way to fuel up first thing, try this: Prepare a package of instant oatmeal and mix in a scoop of whey protein powder and ½ cup of blueberries.

Break the skipping-meals habit. This one's easy. Simply spread your calories out into three meals of about 500 calories each, and two snacks of 100 to 200 calories each, says Liz Applegate, Ph.D., director of sports nutrition at the University of California at Davis. Most men who are trying to lose weight still need at least 1,800 to 2,200 calories a day. Even more important, change your mindset, she says. Think *I'm going to start a new routine,* not *I'm going to restrict myself.* Restriction ultimately leads to really bad moods and then to overeating. And then to worse moods. Look at this effort as a positive, not a negative.

Ditch the I-have-no-time excuse. Sometimes you'd like to eat but you just can't find the time to make a feta-cheese-and-spinach omelet with sweet potato home fries. Been there? Then keep a meal replacement shake on hand. No, it doesn't taste as good as eggs and taters with hot sauce, but it's a smart quickie option. In studies, obesity researchers have found that regularly drinking meal replacements increased a man's chances of losing weight and keeping it off for longer than a year. Aren't nutrition researchers wonderful people? There you go: no more excuses for skipping meals. You can purchase bottled meal replacement shakes that contain various amounts of protein, carbs, fats, vitamins, minerals, even fiber and omega-3s so you can tailor your snack or meal to your specific needs. To save money, you can make these shakes yourself. Here's one recipe designed to replace a meal because it contains about 25 percent calories from protein, 25 percent from fat, and 50 percent from carbohydrate. Very tasty. You'll see.

THE STRAWBERRY POWER BLAST

BLEND TOGETHER:

- 1 cup low-fat vanilla yogurt
- 1 cup 1% milk
- 2 teaspoons peanut butter
- 1 banana
- 1½ cups frozen unsweetened strawberries
- 2 teaspoons sugar
- 2 or 3 large ice cubes

Mix in a blender on high speed until smooth. Drink immediately. Each serving provides 608 calories, 25 grams of protein, 106 grams of carbohydrate, and 11 grams of fat.

FLAB HABIT #2
SPEED-EATING

Life is not a race. Take time to smell the rosemary-shallot confit on red snapper. Chew slowly. Don't inhale. Use the nondiet approach to weight loss: You're not denying yourself food, you're just eating it more slowly. Savoring it. Allowing your body some time so you don't keep eating when you're full, consuming extra calories that your body doesn't need.

In an experiment in the *Journal of Clinical Endocrinology & Metabolism*, 17 healthy men ate $1\frac{1}{4}$ cups of ice cream. They either engulfed it in 5 minutes or took half an hour to savor it. According to study author Alexander Kokkinos, M.D., Ph.D., levels of fullness-causing hormones (known as PYY and GLP-1), which signal the brain to stop eating, were higher among the 30-minute men. In real life, the fast eaters wouldn't feel as full and could be moving on to another course. This is also more reason to avoid starving yourself all day until you are famished at mealtime. When you are starving, you eat faster. Think of the last time you went without eating all day and then sat down in front of a cheese pizza. Our point exactly.

Break the speed-eating habit. Your body is trying to tell you something, so give it a chance. Slow down, chew your food, and savor the flavors. Thoroughly chewing your food increases what researchers call "oro-sensory factors," which send satiation signals to your brain, helping you feel full on less food, according to a 2009 study by Dutch researchers. Study participants who chewed each bite for an extra 3 seconds ended up consuming less. Skip those calorie-clogged smoothies from the juice joint. They go down too quickly and leave you hungry even though they are loaded with energy.

Extra-Value Deal
THE WEIGHT-LOSS "SOLUTION"

It's water. Plain and simple. Here's why: Think of your stomach as a balloon. As you eat, it stretches. And once it expands to its maximum capacity, the sensors throughout your digestive system tell your brain's amygdala that it's time to stop chowing down—regardless of what you've filled your belly with. As Alan Aragon, M.S., *Men's Health*'s nutrition advisor, puts it, "Eating half a roll of toilet paper would make you feel full." To stretch your stomach without stuffing it with calories (or paper products), you need water. Aragon recommends drinking a glass 30 minutes before a meal and sipping frequently while eating. Water-rich foods—soup, salad, fruit, and vegetables—will also fill your belly without contributing excessive calories.

FLAB HABIT #3
PIGGING OUT ON WEEKENDS

You've been good all week long. You've worked hard. You deserve to kick back and unloosen that belt buckle.

You have to change your attitude toward rewards. Sure, you deserve to treat yourself, but it doesn't have to be with an all-you-can-eat buffet. In fact, rewarding yourself with meals just reinforces food's grip on you. And from a practical standpoint, weekend feasts can cause trouble beyond Sunday. In a recent study in the *Journal of Clinical Investigation*, researchers used rats to examine the effects of palmitic acid on leptin, a hormone that regulates appetite. Palmitic acid is found in saturated fat, an ingredient that is often featured in your favorite weekend grub. (Yes, modest amounts of fats can reduce cravings, but weekend pig-outs are rarely modest in the fat category.) "We found that within 3 days, the saturated fat blunts or blocks the ability of leptin to regulate food intake and body weight," says study author Deborah Clegg, Ph.D., of the University of Texas Southwestern Medical Center. So a Friday to Sunday of burgers, fries, beer, and wings may prime your brain to overeat on Monday.

Break the weekend-pig-out habit. You don't have to go cold turkey (though turkey on whole wheat is always smart). Clegg says that your reward for a healthy week of eating should be one cheat meal, not an entire weekend of them. After all, having an all-you-can-eat weekend is like eating poorly for nearly 30 percent of your week. That means you'd be eating well just 70 percent of the time. We call that a C minus. Do you really want below-average results?

Turn your meals upside down. Another extremely effective strategy for beating the overindulgence habit is to rethink the hierarchy of a few of your biggest meals. Instead of building a meal round the meat, think of the meat protein as a garnish. Make your protein a supporting actor to the star vegetables. This is a terrific way to gain some of the benefits of vegetarian eating without actually becoming a vegetarian. If you think about it, this approach is embedded in some of the oldest (and finest) culinary traditions—Japanese, Indian, Chinese, Italian.

FLAB HABIT #4
GORGING ON SALTY SNACKS

Sodium is insidious—it causes us to eat unconsciously. It adds up fast: popcorn at the movies, chips during the game, peanuts at the bar.

Break the salty-snack habit. Salt cravings go away after a couple of weeks on a reduced-salt diet, says Thomas Moore, M.D., an associate provost at Boston University Medical Center. Not many men can replace their go-to snacks with carrots or celery, but give these veg a try: The crunch may be what you crave. Otherwise, try eating small amounts of low-sodium chips and pretzels. Some pretzels have 450 milligrams of

Sneaky Salt Sources

Nine out of 10 Americans exceed their recommended daily sodium limit, a recent survey by the Centers for Disease Control and Prevention found. To cut down, check the labels of processed foods in the categories where sodium tends to lurk.

U.S. RDA of sodium (2,000-calorie diet):
2,400 mg

Average amount of salt consumed per day:
3,466 mg

THE BREAKDOWN:

Grains, breads, cakes, cookies, crackers: **38%**

Meats, poultry, fish, lunch meats, bacon: **28%**

Vegetables, soups, fries, chips **12%**

Milk products: **8%**

Salad dressings, fats: **4%**

Sweets, beverages: **4%**

Legumes, nuts, seeds: **3%**

Eggs: **3%**

sodium per serving, almost 20 percent of your daily intake. Switching to, say, Triscuits, can make a significant dent in that; they have only about 135 milligrams of sodium per serving.

Other ideas. If potato chips are your go-to junk food, try a nutritious root vegetable replacement. Slice root vegetables—parsnips, carrots, sweet potatoes, and beets—very thinly and toss them with olive oil, a pinch of sea salt, and pepper. Roast in a 400°F oven until lightly browned and crispy. If popcorn is your weakness, stay away from supermarket bags and movie theater boxes, which are loaded with calories, sodium, and even trans fats. Pop your own: ¼ cup of kernels in a microwavable bag along with a few teaspoons of vegetable oil and whatever spices you like. Try curry powder, chili powder, and herbs like thyme, rosemary, and oregano. Microwave on high until there are a few seconds between pops.

Then, as you're cooking a dish, skip the salt and, if you want, add just a dash at the table. Why? Because salt added to the surface of a food item is far more noticeable than the same amount of salt cooked into a recipe. A slow reduction of your salt habit pays off in fewer cravings.

Extra-Value Deal
A GRAPEFRUIT APPETIZER?
Maybe you eat less because nothing tastes great after you've eaten a tart grapefruit. Researchers at the Scripps Clinic in San Diego say that people who ate half a grapefruit with every meal lost an average of 3.6 pounds over 12 weeks.

DRINKING SUGARY LIQUIDS

Not all calories require chewing. Everyone knows this, but it's easy to forget just how high in calories liquids can be. They go down so easy. They don't combat hunger. How bad can they be? Plenty. In one study, people were given food in both liquid and sold forms. On days when they ate food in liquid form, they consumed many more calories than when they ate solid food.

Sugary drinks are the leading source of calories in the average American's diet, accounting for nearly 10 percent of calories consumed every day. It's easy to fathom when you consider that a 12-ounce can of soda contains roughly 12 teaspoons of high-fructose corn syrup. And who drinks 12-ouncers anymore? We like our biggie fast-food restaurant drinks—42 ounces of sugary deliciousness (delivering 400-plus calories). History lesson: When McDonald's first opened, a soda was 7 ounces.

Break the liquid lunch habit. Switch from sugary sodas and fruit drinks to water and unsweetened iced teas. It takes a bit of willpower, but the calorie savings can be substantial, especially if you down several cans of pop a day. Natural fruit juices are another sneaky fattener. They sound healthy but they are loaded with calories. A 16-ounce bottle of cranberry-grape juice blend, for instance, contains about 275 calories. Try this: Store half in a jar in the fridge. Refill the bottle with water. You'll make the drink refreshingly tasty—not overly sweet—and you'll be cutting the calories in half.

A Pitcher of Health

Regular soft drinks are now the number-one beverage in America, according to the USDA. Unfortunately, these drinks are loading our diets with empty calories that pack on pounds. Recently, a six-person committee of public-health and nutrition scientists—the Beverage Guidance Panel—created a visual plan for the drinking man. Here's what they suggest for beverage consumption for a person on a 2,200-calorie diet and assuming at least 98 ounces of total fluid per day.

Water: **50 ounces**

Unsweetened tea or coffee: **up to 28 ounces**

Low fat milk: **up to 16 ounces**

Fruit juice (or alcohol): **up to 4 ounces**

FLAB HABIT #6
DRINKING ALCOHOL

Alcohol—beer, wine, mixed drinks, shots—has a distinct association with fat in the midsection. Why? Because when you drink alcohol, your liver burns the alcohol instead of fat. What's more, many alcoholic beverages—especially beer and the sugary sweet cocktails—are very high in calories. It's easy to consume two or three or even four in an evening and end up swallowing more than 700 calories. And that's before the nachos. Here's an exercise to start tonight: Write down how much beer, wine, and other drinks you consume in a week. (Use that cocktail napkin.) You may surprise yourself. Calculate the calories and expect another surprise. A reasonable-sounding two beers a night can mean way more than 2,000 calories a week—almost

an extra day's worth. It can take more than 2 hours of running to burn that off. You call that a weight-loss plan? Besides the empty calories, booze undermines your willpower, says Dawn Jackson Blatner, R.D., spokeswoman for the American Dietetic Association. Which leads to impulse orders of, say, Philly cheese steaks and buffalo wings.

Break the booze habit. Try quitting—for just a week. Check your weight and how your pants fit. Even just 1 week without a drink can have a dramatic impact on your weight. When the week's over, have a celebratory drink, but see if you can live on less. Chances are you'll find the willpower to dramatically cut back. When you do drink, switch to lower-carbohydrate dry red wine (about 4 grams of carbohydrates compared with almost 13 in a regular beer) or low-carb beer.

FLAB HABIT #7
EATING IN FRONT OF THE TV, THEN DOZING OFF

It's a double whammy with a twist. You ingest calories while burning none, and sabotage your secret weight-loss weapon: sleep. Research confirms that people who eat in front of the tube consume more

---

Extra-Value Deal
EAT RIGHT FOR SHORT WORKOUTS

If you're exercising for an hour or less, you don't need to make special dietary accommodations. But you still need to sustain yourself. Eat a meal with at least 200 calories, 20 grams of protein, and 30 grams of carbohydrates an hour or two before a workout. A simple grilled-chicken sandwich will suffice.

calories (nearly 300, in one study) than those who don't, and that the more TV they watch, the less active they are. And researchers at the University of Chicago found that people who lost 3 hours of sleep ate about 200 more calories the next day in snacks than those who slept 8½ hours.

Break the habit that leads to couch pouch. Be active while watching TV. Do some situps and pushups or stretching while catching a show. Or make TV a reward for a workout. And make your DVR earn its keep so you can go to bed on a regular schedule. Sleep is a fine habit when done correctly.

FLAB HABIT #8
NOT EATING ENOUGH VEGETABLES

Tired of hearing this? Well, sorry, we're going to repeat it because this works: Eating lots of vegetables will automatically cause you to lose weight because they are high in water and fiber, which fill you up, and low in calories. Did you know that only 20 percent of men eat the recommended five daily servings of vegetables and fruits? Chances are good that you are a member of the 80 percent team.

Break the anti-vegetable habit. If your meat-to-vegetable ratio is more like 70:30, try flipping that around. How? Loaded salads. Take some green leaves (spinach, red or green leaf lettuce, or romaine lettuce) as a base and dump in baby carrots, broccoli or cauliflower florets, cut-up yellow bell peppers, grape tomatoes, etc. Suddenly you have a full-on vegetarian meal that will satisfy your manly hunger. If 70:30 veg-to-meat is too extreme for you for starters—or the math is too hard—

here's an even simpler way to ensure that you are eating more vegetables and fruits every day at every meal: Draw an imaginary line down the middle of your plate. Fill half with vegetables or fruit, the other half with protein. Eat the produce half first. Chances are you won't finish the meat half because you'll already feel full.

FLAB HABIT #9
MINDLESS EATING

What do you do when you are sitting in the kitchen next to a big bowl of chips or M&Ms? You dig in even if you aren't hungry. It's the see-food-eat-food conundrum that leads to mindless eating. The food is front and center, and your hands and mouth need something to do. Mindless eating is the downfall of many attempting to lose weight because it's so hard to avoid and very difficult to quantify. You don't remember how much you ate because you're eating without thinking. Cornell University researchers studied this phenomenon and found this simple truth: We are more likely to eat the first food we see than the fifth food. "We are masters of our own demise," says study researcher Brian Wansink, Ph.D., author of *Mindless Eating: Why We Eat More Than We Think.*

Break the habit of eating without thinking. The first step is to delay that automatic reach for the food, and it's crucial. If you can pause just a few seconds, you can remind yourself to think about what you are poised to do. It'll give you a chance to ask yourself, "Am I really hungry?" If you're not really hungry, it's your mind and muscle memory playing tricks on you. You reach for the bowl of chips because that's just what your mind tells you you're supposed to do when you see one. But by pausing, you are able to make the next critical step: distracting yourself by changing your environment. Move to another room away from the food, or drop and do 10 pushups. Or try this yoga breathing trick: Inhale while counting slowly to five; exhale and count slowly to five; repeat three to five times before eating. A study in the *Journal of the American Dietetic Association* shows that yoga increases mindful eating and results in less weight gain over time.

To avoid the temptation in the first place, hide your snacks. Remember that Cornell study: The first food you see—the food that's closest—will be the one you eat. So hide your chips, candy, sugary drinks, cookies, and other snacks in the basement, in a high, hard-to-reach cabinet; make yourself work to get to them, and you'll be less likely to eat them. Replace that chip

Extra-Value Deal
HEAT UP YOUR METABOLISM
Several studies have shown that eating a spicy meal can boost your metabolism by up to 25 percent and keep the elevated calorie burning going for up to 3 hours. Add jalapeño, habanero, or cayenne peppers to your meals. Capsaicin, the chemical in peppers that gives them their bite, works by speeding up your heart rate. Another way do to the same without burning your tongue? Have a cup of green tea. The caffeine and a chemical in green tea called EGCG combine to speed up your heart rate and cause your nervous system to run quicker, helping you burn more calories.

bowl with a bowl of fresh apples. Even better than hiding your snacks is eliminating them from your home. If they aren't there, you can't eat them, right? Clean out your cupboard and fridge, then restock them with almonds and other nuts to snack on, cheese, fruits and vegetables, and canned tuna, chicken, and salmon. You can do the same at work. Sneak a small refrigerator into your office. Stock it with healthy snacks and you'll be far less likely to find yourself at the doughnut shop drive-thru or the vending machine.

FLAB HABIT #10
EATING OUT OFTEN
How many times do you eat food outside of your kitchen; that is, food prepared by someone who you don't know? If you kept a food journal like the one on page 65, you'd know exactly. Once a day? Twice? More than 14 meals at take-out or sit-down restaurants in a week? It's pretty easy to do. Therein lies the problem: Eating out is easy. It's convenient. You don't have dishes to wash. But it's also the quickest way to put on unwanted pounds. Consider this: One study found that people consume up to 500 more calories per day when they eat at restaurants compared with when they prepare their own meals at home. Think about it: Cook seven meals at home instead of eating at restaurants and you could save 3,500 calories per week. That's equivalent to a pound of fat.

One of the reasons that restaurant fare is so bad for our bellies is that when we eat out, we shovel more food in. It's not uncommon to find that restaurant portions are triple the amount of food that you need to feel satisfied. Portion sizes have grown dramatically since the late 1950s when, for example, a hamburger held an ounce of ground beef between the buns (today it's 6 ounces or more), breakfast muffins weighed 1½ ounces (today they are typically 8 ounces, packing 400 calories), and a large soda measured 8 fluid ounces versus 32 ounces today.

Break the fast-food habit. Eating at a nice restaurant or grabbing a great sandwich for lunch—those are joys you shouldn't deny yourself. And you don't have to. Not if you cut out those processed fast-food meals that are among the most unhealthy, laden with calories, preservatives, sodium, and fat. Breaking the fast-food habit means changing behaviors and becoming more aware of the choke hold of snacking. Our appetite for snacks has become insatiable. Between 1977 and 2006, Americans' snacking increased 11 percent while our average downtime between meals dropped from 4½ hours to 3½ hours, according to a 2009 study in the *American Journal of Clinical Nutrition.* The fast-food chains couldn't be happier with our snack fetish. McDonald's hawks a 340-calorie Snack Wrap, and Taco Bell's "FourthMeal" campaign encourages eaters to inflate the midnight snack into a full-fledged second dinner, complete with its 790-calorie Nachos BellGrande.

The easiest way to stop making impulsive turns into the fast-food drive-thru is to make sure you're eating satiety-inducing nutrients at every meal. Doing so will reduce your urge for food between meals. How do you ensure your belly is filled with satisfying food? Prepare your meals yourself. Do it gradually. If you chow down at fast-food joints five times a week, dial back to one or two. Get into the habit of grocery shopping and meal planning, preparing more of your meals—even lunches—at home. And not only will you shed pounds quickly, you'll carve lots of dough off your food bill. You can find yourself saving hundreds of dollars every month. And that'll motivate you to cook at home—and save—even more.

Also: If you must snack, make sure you have snack-sized hunger satisfiers at the ready. Grab food that's high in protein or fiber, like beef jerky, nuts, or cottage cheese, and keep your consumption under 200 calories. Two-hundred calories is key. That's enough food to keep gut gurgling at bay without packing in a mini-meal. Whatever you do, skip the processed snacks that prime your gut for more, more, more. It's how a doughnut leads to a growling stomach before lunch. It's how a drive-thru dinner can lead to FourthMeal at midnight. And it's how you can eat all day and never feel full.

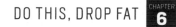

ACTION PLAN

KEEP A FOOD JOURNAL

Recording your food intake serves two purposes: It gives you a clear picture of the food you're eating, what kind, when, and the circumstances that may affect the amount you're eating. Second, it helps you to become hyper-aware of what you are putting in your mouth. Sometimes just knowing that you will create a record of your indulgence can give you the willpower to put down that doughnut. Keep track of what you eat and drink for at least 3 days—preferably a week. The picture of your daily plate will emerge very quickly and poignantly.

DATE: _____

MEAL	FOOD/DRINK (# OF SERVINGS)	HOW MUCH?	CIRCUMSTANCES
Breakfast			
Lunch			
Dinner			
Snacks			

8-ounce glasses of water: ○ ○ ○ ○ ○ ○ ○ ○

DATE: _____

MEAL	FOOD/DRINK (# OF SERVINGS)	HOW MUCH?	CIRCUMSTANCES
Breakfast			
Lunch			
Dinner			
Snacks			

8-ounce glasses of water: ◯ ◯ ◯ ◯ ◯ ◯ ◯ ◯

DATE: _____

MEAL	FOOD/DRINK (# OF SERVINGS)	HOW MUCH?	CIRCUMSTANCES
Breakfast			
Lunch			
Dinner			
Snacks			

8-ounce glasses of water: ◯ ◯ ◯ ◯ ◯ ◯ ◯ ◯

DATE: _____

MEAL	FOOD/DRINK (# OF SERVINGS)	HOW MUCH?	CIRCUMSTANCES
Breakfast			
Lunch			
Dinner			
Snacks			

8-ounce glasses of water: ◯ ◯ ◯ ◯ ◯ ◯ ◯ ◯

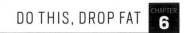

DATE: _____

MEAL	FOOD/DRINK (# OF SERVINGS)	HOW MUCH?	CIRCUMSTANCES
Breakfast			
Lunch			
Dinner			
Snacks			

8-ounce glasses of water: ◯ ◯ ◯ ◯ ◯ ◯ ◯ ◯

DATE: _____

MEAL	FOOD/DRINK (# OF SERVINGS)	HOW MUCH?	CIRCUMSTANCES
Breakfast			
Lunch			
Dinner			
Snacks			

8-ounce glasses of water: ◯ ◯ ◯ ◯ ◯ ◯ ◯ ◯

DATE: _____

MEAL	FOOD/DRINK (# OF SERVINGS)	HOW MUCH?	CIRCUMSTANCES
Breakfast			
Lunch			
Dinner			
Snacks			

8-ounce glasses of water: ◯ ◯ ◯ ◯ ◯ ◯ ◯ ◯

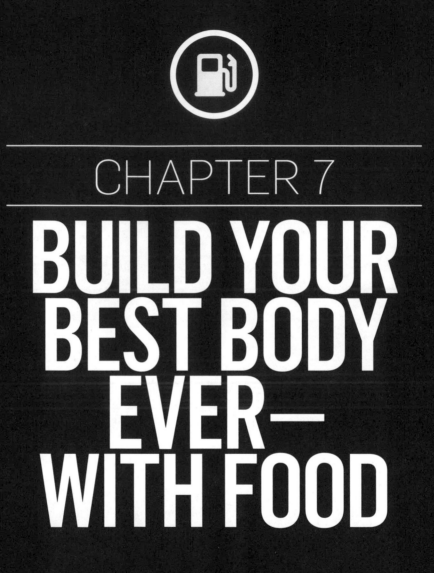

CHAPTER 7

BUILD YOUR BEST BODY EVER— WITH FOOD

In this chapter, we will focus on nutritional strategies
that will foster the muscle-rebuilding process so that it works
optimally. We'll provide a list of nine important foods for
muscle growth. By adding these ingredients to your diet,
you will ensure that you pack your body with everything it
needs to build lean, hard muscle and lots of it. We'll also offer
optimum refueling strategies, advice on how to eat to burn
fat, energize your workouts, and boost your endurance.
This information is as critical—maybe even more important—
to building muscle as the workout chapters later in the book.
Don't discount the power of food to reach your muscle goals.
So put down that dumbbell and grab a grocery list.

One thing that you should get through your head and make peace with: To make more muscle, you're going to have to eat more food. A guy who weighs about 175 pounds and is looking to gain muscle, for example, will end up eating about 400 calories more per day. Maybe even 500. You need these extra calories to energize your exercise. Plus, you'll need more energy to rebuild the muscle that you've broken down through hefting weights. Protein, as you know, helps repair muscle tissue damaged by resistance training. It's also loaded with the amino acids your body needs to make the hormones and enzymes required for the production of red blood cells and the strength of your immune system.

HOW MUCH PROTEIN IS ENOUGH?

Think big. Most adults would benefit from eating more than the recommended daily intake of 56 grams, says Donald Layman, Ph.D., a professor emeritus of nutrition at the University of Illinois. The benefit goes beyond muscles, he says: Protein dulls hunger and can help prevent obesity, diabetes, and heart disease. How much do you need? Step on a scale and be honest with yourself about your workout regimen. According to Mark Tarnopolsky, M.D., Ph.D., who studies exercise and nutrition at McMaster University in Hamilton, Ontario, highly trained athletes thrive on 0.77 gram of daily protein per pound of body weight. That's 139 grams for a 180-pound man. Men who work out 5 or more days a week for an hour or longer need 0.55 gram per pound. And men who work out 3 to 5 days a week for 45 minutes to an hour need 0.45 gram per pound. So a 180-pound guy who works out regularly needs about 80 grams of protein a day.

Now, if you're trying to lose weight, protein is still crucial. The fewer calories you consume, the more calories should come from protein, says Layman. You need to boost your protein intake to between 0.45 and 0.68 gram per pound to preserve calorie-burning muscle mass. And no, that extra protein won't wreck your kidneys: "Taking in more than the recommended dose won't confer more benefit. It won't hurt you, but you'll just burn it off as extra energy," Dr. Tarnopolsky says.

All protein is not the same. Many foods, including nuts and beans, can provide a good dose of protein. But the best sources are dairy products, eggs, meat, and fish, Layman says. Animal protein is complete—it contains the right proportions of the essential amino acids your body can't synthesize on its own. It's possible to build complete protein from plant-based foods by combining legumes, nuts, and grains at one meal or over the course of a day. But you'll need to eat 20 to 25 percent more plant-based protein to reap the same benefits animal sources provide, says Dr. Tarnopolsky.

So if protein can help keep weight off, is a chicken wing dipped in blue-cheese dressing a diet secret? Not quite: Total calories still count. Scale down your fat and carbohydrate intake to make room for lean protein: eggs, low-fat milk, yogurt, lean meat, and fish. But remember, if you're struggling with your weight, fat itself is not the culprit; carbs are the likely problem. Fat will help keep you full, while carbs can put you on a blood-sugar roller coaster that leaves you hungry later.

THE LIST

THE LIST: 9 ESSENTIAL MUSCLE FOODS

EGGS: THE PERFECT PROTEIN

The protein in eggs has the highest biological value—a measure of how well it supports your body's protein needs—of any food, including our beloved beef. "Calorie for calorie, you need less protein from eggs than you do from other sources to achieve the same muscle building," says Jeff Volek, Ph.D., R.D., an exercise and nutrition researcher at the University of Connecticut. But you have to eat the yolk. In addition to protein, it also contains vitamin B_{12}, which is necessary for fat breakdown and muscle contraction. (And no, eating a few eggs a day won't increase your risk of heart disease.) Eggs are vitamins and minerals over easy; they're packed with riboflavin, folate, vitamins B_6, B_{12}, D, and E, and iron, phosphorus, and zinc.

ALMONDS: MUSCLE MEDICINE

Crunch for crunch, almonds are one of the best sources of alpha-tocopherol vitamin E—the form that's best absorbed by your body. That matters to your muscles because "vitamin E is a potent antioxidant that can help prevent free-radical damage after heavy workouts," says Volek. And the fewer hits taken from free radicals, the faster your muscles will recover from a

workout and start growing. How many almonds should you munch? Two handfuls a day should do it. A Toronto University study found that men can eat this amount daily without gaining any weight. Almonds double as brain insurance. A recent study published in the *Journal of the American Medical Association* found that those men who consumed the most vitamin E—from food sources, not supplements—had a 67 percent lower risk of Alzheimer's disease than those eating the least vitamin E.

SALMON: THE GROWTH REGULATOR

It's swimming with high-quality protein and omega-3 fatty acids. "Omega-3s can decrease muscle-protein breakdown after your workout, improving recovery," says Tom Incledon, R.D., a nutritionist with Human Performance Specialists. This is important, because to build muscle you need to store new protein faster than your body breaks down the old stuff. Order some salmon jerky from www.freshseafood.com. It'll keep forever in your gym bag and tastes mighty close to cold-smoked cow. Omega-3s offer another benefit: They'll reduce your risk of heart disease and diabetes. Researchers at Louisiana State University found that when overweight people added 1.8 grams of DHA—an omega-3 fatty acid in fish oil—to their daily diets, their insulin resistance decreased by 70 percent in 12 weeks.

YOGURT: THE GOLDEN RATIO

Even with the aura of estrogen surrounding it, "yogurt is an ideal combination of protein and carbohydrates for exercise recovery and muscle growth," says Doug Kalman, Ph.D, R.D., director of nutrition at Miami Research Associates. Buy Greek yogurt, which has double the protein of regular yogurt. If you prefer regular, avoid the sugar-free yogurts and buy yogurt with fruit buried at the bottom.

How Much Protein Should You Eat?

Your body needs protein to repair and create skin, organ, and muscle cells. How much you need depends on how often and intensely you're damaging those cells through exercise, says nutritionist Cassandra Forsythe, Ph.D., R.D.

GENERAL PROTEIN RECOMMENDATIONS BASED ON ACTIVITY	GRAMS PER POUND OF BODY WEIGHT
Sedentary adults	0.4 g/lb
Recreational athletes	0.5 g/lb
Strength athletes	0.5–0.9 g/lb*
Endurance athletes	0.5–0.6 g/lb
Ultra-endurance athletes	0.5–0.9 g/lb

*Not all experts agree
Source: *Nutrition for Sport and Exercise*, 2nd edition

The extra carbohydrates from the fruit will boost your blood levels of insulin, one of the keys to reducing postexercise protein breakdown. Yogurt is also rich in CLA (conjugated linoleic acid), a special type of fat shown in some studies to reduce body fat.

BEEF: CARVABLE CREATINE

More than just a piece of charbroiled protein, beef is also a major source of iron and zinc, two crucial muscle-building nutrients. Plus, it's the number-one food source of creatine—your body's energy supply for pumping iron—2 grams for every 16 ounces. For maximum muscle with minimum calories, look for "rounds" or "loins"—butcherspeak for meat cuts that are extra-lean. Or check out the new "flat iron" cut. It's very lean and the second most tender cut of beef overall.

OLIVE OIL: LIQUID ENERGY

Sure, you could oil up your chest and arms and strike a pose, but it works better if you eat the stuff. "The monounsaturated fat in olive oil appears to act as an anti-catabolic nutrient," says Kalman. In other words, it prevents muscle breakdown by lowering levels of a sinister cellular protein called tumor necrosis factor-alpha, which is linked with muscle wasting and weakness (kind of like what happens when you watch *The View*). And while all olive oil is high in monounsaturated fats, try to use the extra-virgin variety whenever possible; it has a higher level of free-radical-fighting vitamin E than the less chaste stuff. Olive oil and monounsaturated fats also boast other health benefits, having been associated

TIME FOR YOUR
PROTEIN INFUSION

EVERY TIME YOU EAT at least 30 grams of protein, you trigger a burst of protein synthesis that lasts about 3 hours. But think about it: When do you eat most of your protein? At dinner, right? That means you could be fueling muscle growth for only a few hours a day, and breaking down muscle the rest of the time. Instead, you should spread out your protein intake throughout the day. Your body can process only so much protein in a single sitting. A recent study from the University of Texas found that consuming 90 grams of protein at one meal provides the same benefit as eating 30 grams. It's like a gas tank, says study author Douglas Paddon-Jones, Ph.D.: "There's only so much you can put in to maximize performance; the rest is spill-over." Eating protein at all three meals—plus snacking two or three times a day on proteins such as cheese, jerky, and milk—will help you eat less overall. People who start the day with a protein-rich breakfast consume 200 fewer calories a day than those who chow down on a carbohydrate-heavy breakfast, like a jam-smeared bagel.

Every guy in the gym knows he should consume some protein after a workout. But how much and when? "When you work out, your muscles are primed to respond to protein, and you have a window of opportunity to promote muscle growth," says exercise and nutrition researcher Jeff Volek, Ph.D., R.D. Volek recommends splitting your dose of protein, eating half 30 minutes before the workout and the other half 30 minutes after. A total of 10 to 20 grams of protein is ideal, he says. And wrap a piece of bread around that turkey, because carbs can raise insulin; this slows protein breakdown, which speeds muscle growth after your workout. Moreover, you won't use your stored protein for energy; you'll rely instead on the carbs to replenish you. One study, published in the *American Journal of Clinical Nutrition*, pinpointed 20 grams as the best amount of postworkout protein to maximize muscle growth. You're doing this because resistance exercise breaks down muscle. This requires a fresh infusion of amino acids to repair and build it. "If you're lifting weights and you don't consume protein, it's almost counterproductive," says Volek. Protein also helps build enzymes that allow your body to adapt to endurance sports like running and biking.

with everything from lower rates of heart disease and colon cancer to a reduced risk of diabetes and osteoporosis.

WATER: THE MUSCLE BATH

Whether it's in your shins or your shoulders, muscle is approximately 80 percent water. "Even a change of as little as 1 percent in body water can impair exercise performance and adversely affect recovery," says Volek. For example, a 1997 German study found that protein synthesis occurs at a higher rate in muscle cells that are well hydrated, compared with dehydrated cells. English translation: The more parched you are, the slower your body uses

Secrets of the Muscle Pro

For nearly 20 years, California-based nutritionist Alan Aragon, M.S., has analyzed the latest research on food, supplements, and training in order to help pro athletes and average guys hit their weight goals. Here are the things *he* does to stay in top condition.

1. **How I supplement my diet.** "I eat healthy, but to cover any gaps I take a daily Kirkland Signature multi. Kirkland is verified by the USP (United States Pharmacopeia), so I trust the label. I also take 1.2 grams of omega-3s (EPA/DHA) and 200 milligrams of magnesium citrate because it's often underdosed in multivitamins."

2. **How I nourish my muscles.** "I aim for 1 gram of protein per pound of lean body mass. You can also use your target body weight: For example, if you're 200 pounds and want to be 180, then eat 180 grams of protein a day. I eat roughly 90 grams from food and 90 grams from a four-scoop shake. I mix Now brand whey protein isolate with Gaspari MyoFusion."

3. **How I build strength fast.** "I weight-train for an hour 4 days a week, alternating upper-body and lower-body days. My objective is to rest as little as necessary between sets and still maintain my lifting poundages and repetition targets. This makes my workout more efficient; plus, it delivers cardio benefits. I typically do 2 sets of 10 to 12 exercises, broken into complementary pairings of muscle groups—for instance, bench press [chest] and barbell rows [back] or leg extensions [quads] and leg curls [hamstrings/glutes]."

4. **How I snack without guilt.** "I eat 10 percent of my daily calories from any source. That means 250 calories from a small bowl of fudge ice cream or two glasses of cabernet. When I design diets, there's always leeway for 'wild card' calories. Research shows that flexible eaters are more likely to hit their weight targets in the long term than people who are more rigid."

5. **How I power up.** "I make a three-egg omelet with $1/3$ cup of Parmesan, two sliced green chile peppers, and six grape tomatoes, and I have chicken sausage on the side. I top it all with kimchi—spicy Korean pickled cabbage."

protein to build muscle. A 2008 study in the *Journal of Applied Physiology* found that dehydrated lifters produced more stress hormones, including cortisol, while reducing the release of testosterone, the body's best muscle builder. Not sure how dry you are? "Weigh yourself before and after each exercise session. Then drink 24 ounces of water for every pound lost," says Larry Kenney, Ph.D., a physiology researcher at Pennsylvania State University. Internal soaking is also good for your most important muscle, your heart. Researchers at Loma Linda University found that men who drank five or more 8-ounce glasses of water a day were 54 percent less likely to suffer a fatal heart attack than those who drank two or fewer.

CAFFEINE: THE REPETITION BUILDER

Fueling your workout with caffeine will help you lift longer. A recent study published in *Medicine & Science in Sports & Exercise* found that men who drank 2½ cups of coffee a few hours before an exercise test were able to sprint 9 percent longer than when they didn't drink any. (It's believed the caffeine directly stimulates the muscles.) And since sprinting and weight lifting are both anaerobic activities—exercises that don't require oxygen—a jolt of joe should help you pump out more reps. (Caution: If you have a history of high blood pressure, don't take caffeine or drink caffeinated drinks. Check with your doctor first.)

PROTEIN SUPPLEMENTS: BUILD MUSCLE WHILE SLEEPING

Anyone can benefit from the quick hit of amino acids provided by a protein supplement, bar, or shake. They provide a fast way to consume a lot of protein and calories without the saturated fat and cholesterol found in protein-rich whole foods like beef and eggs. What's more, they are convenient. When you don't have the luxury of grilling a chicken breast or scrambling eggs, you can get your protein fix in a handy meal-replacement bar or in a shaker bottle with a couple of scoops of protein powder in water.

Your best bet for a postworkout protein hit is a fast-absorbing, high-quality protein like whey protein powder (derived from milk): "It appears in your bloodstream 15 minutes after you consume it," Volek says. Whey protein is also the best source of leucine, an amino acid that behaves more like a hormone in your body: "It's more than a building block of protein—it actually activates protein synthesis," Volek says. Whey contains 10 percent leucine while other animal-based proteins have as little as 5 percent. Casein, another milk protein sold in supplement form, provides a slower-absorbing but more sustained source of amino acids, making it a great choice for a snack before you hit the sack. "Casein should help you maintain a positive protein balance during the night," says Volek. Building muscle while you sleep? Thanks to protein supplements, anything's possible.

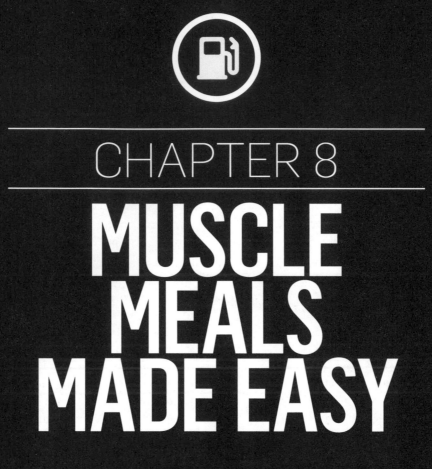

CHAPTER 8

MUSCLE MEALS MADE EASY

You probably have a desert-island list of the music or books—or women—you'd want to have around if you were shipwrecked. But when it comes to the meals you can live on indefinitely, it's not as simple as playing favorites. The best recipes are the ones tailored just for you: foods that fit after a long day at work, when someone stays for breakfast, or late at night when you crave sustenance. Master these dishes and you'll never be stranded, no matter when your hunger strikes.

BIG BREAKFAST FRY-UP

When a woman stays for breakfast, cold cereal won't cut it. But juggling the timing on eggs, bacon, and home fries can be tricky. Use this all-in-one recipe instead. "Because you serve it rustic-style—directly from the pan it was cooked in—it's a simple yet sexy presentation," says chef Tyler Florence of Wayfare Tavern in San Francisco and the author of Tyler Florence Family Meals. *"Add some toasted country bread and you're done."*

6 strips bacon, cut into 1-inch pieces, or 4 quarter-inch-thick slices pancetta, diced

1 cup button mushrooms, quartered

1 cup grape tomatoes, halved

Coarse salt and freshly ground pepper

Extra-virgin olive oil

8 large eggs

Fresh thyme leaves

1 handful of arugula leaves

6 slices Italian country loaf, toasted

1. In a large skillet over medium heat, cook the bacon until crispy, 5 to 6 minutes. Then transfer it to a paper-towel-lined plate to drain, leaving the fat in the pan. Add the mushrooms and tomatoes to the pan and sauté on medium high until the mushrooms are lightly browned, about 1 minute. Sprinkle with salt and pepper and transfer the mixture to a plate.

2. Reduce the heat to low; add 1 to 2 teaspoons of olive oil to the pan if needed, and then carefully crack in the eggs. Cook them sunny-side up, or until the whites are set but the yolks are still runny.

3. Distribute the bacon and the mushroom-tomato mixture evenly around the pan. Sprinkle on salt and pepper, and add the thyme and arugula. Add a drizzle of olive oil. Serve straight from the pan with the toasted bread.

MAKES 4 SERVINGS

No Time? No Worries.

Four Shortcuts to a Fast Meal

When it comes to cooking, time just isn't on your side. In a recent *Men's Health* survey, 37 percent of men said they cook at home at least three times a week, but 48 percent avoid it because it takes too long. To shave precious minutes off your cooking times, use these tips from Mark Bittman, author of *How to Cook Everything*.

1. **Chop everything at once.** Have your vegetables prepped and ready to go before you start cooking in order to avoid slowdowns along the way.

2. **Clean as you go.** You don't have to be obsessive about this, but if you use a pan, wash it; you'll have more space to cook and less to do after you eat.

3. **Multitask.** Make the salad while your meat cooks; have the rice going while you peel the shrimp; grate Parmesan while you wait for the pasta water to boil.

4. **Cook the basics in bulk.** When you cook beans, grains, broth, or tomato sauce, make double and freeze the rest. With a minimum of effort, you'll have a head start on your next meal.

The Weeknight Pasta
LINGUINE WITH CLAMS

Opening a jar of red sauce might be the default move when you're craving pasta, but there's another way to go: quick-cooking clams in a sauce made from pantry staples, such as olive oil and garlic. "It's the easiest way to look like a rock star," says Frank Falcinelli, co-chef at Frankies 457 in Brooklyn. "Grab some clams on your way home from work and you're set," adds Frank Castronovo, the other co-chef at Frankies.

- $1/2$ pound linguine or spaghetti
- 2 tablespoons extra-virgin olive oil
- 2 garlic cloves, smashed and finely chopped
- 1 large pinch red pepper flakes
- 12 littleneck clams, scrubbed
  Coarse salt
- $1/4$ cup finely chopped flat-leaf parsley
  Freshly ground black pepper

1. Bring a large pot of water to a boil, salt it well, and add the pasta. Now start the sauce: Add the olive oil to a large skillet over medium-high heat. After a minute, add the garlic and cook it, stirring, until it's deeply golden but not yet browned, 2 to 3 minutes.

2. Add the red-pepper flakes. Then add the clams, cover the pan, and reduce the heat to medium low. Cook, shaking the pan occasionally, until the clams open and release their juices, about 5 minutes.

3. Take the pasta off the heat a minute or so earlier than the package instructions specify. Drain it well and transfer it to a platter. Pour the clam mixture on top and sprinkle on a pinch of salt and the parsley. Finish with lots of freshly ground pepper.

MAKES 2 SERVINGS

The Late-Night Snack
THE TORTA DOG

After a long night out, it's a shame to quell your hunger by dipping carrots in peanut butter. There's another way to engineer the contents of your fridge into a snack: the Torta Dog. "It's a fast, creative version of a classic Mexican sandwich," says Vinny Dotolo of Animal restaurant in Los Angeles. "It's got the hit of protein you need, and it works no matter what you put on it."

- 1 all-beef hot dog
- 1 soft corn tortilla
  Small handful of shredded Cheddar or Jack cheese
  Your choice of toppings: cooked bacon, canned beans, sliced avocado, sour cream, chopped tomato, salsa, sliced scallions
  Hot sauce or sliced pickled jalapeño chiles to taste

Microwave the hot dog on a plate until warmed, about 30 seconds. Then place it on the tortilla and top it evenly with cheese. Microwave again until the cheese is melted. Add your toppings, fold up the tortilla, and enjoy.

MAKES 1 SERVING

The Fast, Impressive Dinner
POLLO ALLA DIAVOLO

Roasting a chicken has always been a great way to score chef points effortlessly. This version cooks up fast—and looks amazing on a platter. Start a day ahead by marinating the bird. After you roast it, you'll make a quick pan sauce. "We use homemade pickled peppers for the sauce, but store-bought works fine," says Nick Anderer, chef of Maialino in New York City. "The chicken's great with sautéed broccoli rabe or roasted potatoes."

- 3 tablespoons extra-virgin olive oil
- 1 teaspoon coarse salt
- 6 sprigs fresh thyme
  Cracked black pepper to taste
  Red-pepper flakes to taste
- 1 whole chicken (3 to 4 pounds), butterflied (ask the butcher to do this, or use four leg quarters)
- 1 cup low-sodium chicken broth
- 1 cup pickling liquid from jarred hot cherry peppers, plus peppers for serving
- 2 tablespoons tomato sauce or puree

1. The day before you cook the chicken, combine the oil, salt, thyme, pepper, and red-pepper flakes in a wide baking dish. Add the chicken, turning it to coat it evenly, and then cover and refrigerate it overnight.

2. Half an hour before you're ready to cook, remove the chicken from the fridge. Preheat the oven to 375°F. Place a cast-iron skillet or other ovenproof pan in the oven until it's medium hot, about 5 minutes.

3. Remove the pan from the oven and add the chicken, skin side down. Then add another cast-iron skillet on top of the bird to weigh it down. Place the chicken in the oven to roast until it's golden brown and juices run clear when it's pierced in the hip joint, 45 to 55 minutes. Remove the chicken to a cutting board to rest, leaving the juices in the pan.

4. To make the sauce, place the pan on medium-low heat and whisk in the broth, pickling liquid, and tomato sauce, scraping any browned bits from the bottom of the pan. Simmer until the liquid is slightly thickened, 5 to 10 minutes. Cut the chicken into quarters and serve each with the pan sauce and a cherry pepper.

MAKES 4 SERVINGS

The Go-To Stir-Fry
LEMONGRASS PORK WITH BOK CHOY

When you've eaten one too many burgers, you need a hit of vegetables. This Southeast Asian–style stir-fry is easy to make—no need for a superhot wok—and has a fresh taste that they can't match. "For the vegetables, you can use any hearty leafy greens that you have on hand," says Tien Ho, former chef at Má Pêche in New York City.

- 4 tablespoons canola oil
- 1 stalk lemongrass (outer layer discarded), finely chopped
- 2 shallots, finely chopped
- 4 garlic cloves, finely chopped
- 1 pound ground pork
- 1 teaspoon red-pepper flakes
- $\frac{1}{4}$ cup fish sauce (available in the Asian aisle of the supermarket)
  Pinch of salt and sugar
- 1 package (14 ounces) flat rice noodles
- 1 medium onion, halved and thinly sliced
- 2 baby bok choy (bottoms trimmed), thinly sliced crosswise
- 1 bunch Chinese broccoli, sliced
- 1 handful of fresh basil leaves

1. In a medium skillet, heat 2 tablespoons of the canola oil on medium. Add the chopped lemongrass, shallots, and garlic, and sauté the mixture until fragrant, about 2 minutes. Remove the sautéed ingredients to a plate.

2. In the same skillet over medium heat, sauté the ground pork, breaking up any large clumps, until it's cooked through, 5 to 7 minutes. Add the lemongrass mixture, along with the red-pepper flakes, fish sauce, and salt and sugar. Continue to cook until the sauce becomes thickened, about 5 minutes. Remove from the heat and set aside.

3. Cook the rice noodles according to the package instructions. In a large skillet on medium high, heat the remaining 2 tablespoons of canola oil. Then add the onion and cook until slightly soft, about 4 minutes. Add the bok choy and Chinese broccoli, and cook until just tender, about 4 more minutes.

4. Add the pork mixture and rice noodles to the vegetables. Then add the basil and toss to combine, adjusting the seasoning as needed.

MAKES 4 SERVINGS

The Perfect Preworkout Meal

Some people say training on an empty stomach burns more fat: You blow through your glycogen stores in about an hour, and then your body turns to fat stores for energy. The problem with that approach is that your body will soon start to burn muscle tissue as well.

To avoid this, eat a simple yet smart meal beforehand. Your preworkout meal should be relatively low in fat and fiber so it's easily digestible, but not highly glycemic, either—you don't want an insulin spike and a mood crash before you reach the gym. The protein should be easily digested and quickly available.

- The classic is a turkey sandwich. But you have to use the right ingredients. Try high-protein Ezekiel bread, which you can find at health-food stores or bake yourself. It contains wheat, barley, beans, lentils, millet, and spelt (a kind of grain). Add 2 to 3 ounces of fresh-roasted, low-sodium turkey breast (not the salt-laden prepackaged kind), a couple of tomato slices, some bean sprouts for crunch, and honey mustard. (Per sandwich: 300 calories, 30 g protein, 30 g carbohydrates, 10 g fat)

Then, on the way to the gym, down one of the following snacks:

- Handful of raisins and nuts. Raisins give you a simple carb for immediate energy, and nuts give you a little fat and a feeling of satiety. (250 calories, 7 g protein, 30 g carbohydrates)

- Piece of fruit. Apples and plums offer just enough carbs to get you going. (40 calories, 10 g carbohydrates each)

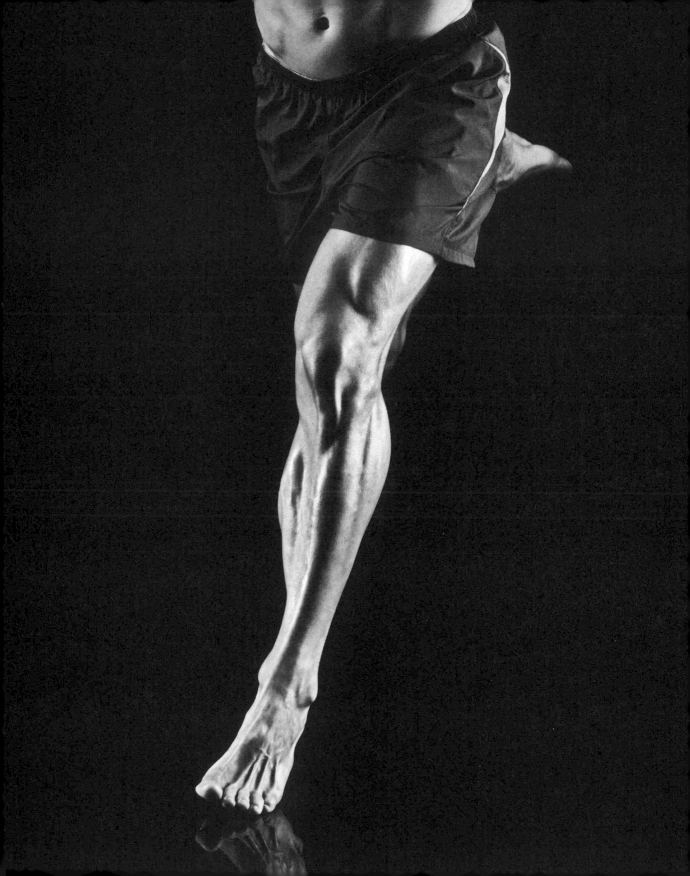

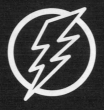

PART THREE

SPEED

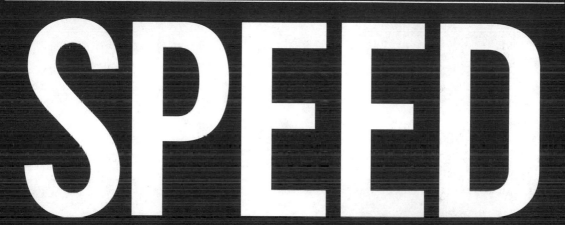

ACCELERATE YOUR
RESULTS AND BECOME
FASTER, MORE FLEXIBLE,
AND MORE EXPLOSIVE
THAN EVER BEFORE

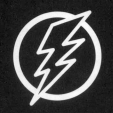

CHAPTER 9

STRETCH FOR STRENGTH

L ack of flexibility is a huge problem for people who are attempting to get back in shape, because they often exercise without first priming their muscles for the stress of all that lifting, running, jumping, and twisting. It's sort of like trying to run your car without oil; the engine will seize up without lubrication. By the same token, if you don't get blood flowing to your muscles, your body won't move as well and you'll risk tearing something. And you'll pay a lot more to an orthopedic surgeon than you would to an auto mechanic! Stretching offers all sorts of benefits. Done right, it prepares your muscles, joints, and connective tissues for your workout. Certain types of moving stretches elevate your core temperature, improve bloodflow to your tissues, and loosen tight muscles and ligaments, and, when performed correctly, can even stabilize the body's critical core of abdominal, lower back, and gluteal muscles that are engaged in nearly every movement you make. Improving your flexibility can also boost your strength, according to a study in the journal *Medicine & Science in Sports & Exercise*. How? By increasing your range of motion and lengthening your muscles, which allows you to produce more force and lift more weight. And ultimately, of course, that leads to more muscle, too. Flexibility also is crucial to good overall health and remaining pain free, especially as you get older and your joints lose lubrication, and certainly if, like most of us, you have a desk job, which promotes stiffness and compromises stability.

Now, before we have you start bending over backward, we need to do a little remedial education about stretching. We want you to forget everything you learned about stretching from your high-school gym teacher or track coach. The science of stretching has long been misunderstood, and people have become injured because of the misinformation. First, let's get you educated about the two distinct types of stretching: static and dynamic.

Help for Lower-Back Pain

A few Sun Salutations could help fix a loused-up lumbar region. According to a report in the *Annals of Internal Medicine*, yoga may relieve back pain. Scientists studied 101 back-pain sufferers as they participated weekly in either one 75-minute yoga class or a 75-minute strength-and-stretching class. (Both groups also practiced at home.) After 26 weeks, the yoga students felt less pain and used fewer pain relievers than the exercising group. Researchers believe certain principles unique to viniyoga—the style used in the study—may have made it more effective. "You learn to pay attention to your body, your breathing, and what movements irritate your back," says lead author Karen Sherman, Ph.D. Before you sign up for a yoga class, see a doctor to rule out spine or disk disease.

STATIC STRETCHING

You've probably done static stretching most of your life. A good example of a static stretch is the classic hamstring stretch in which you lean forward until you feel a slight discomfort in your hamstrings, then hold that position for a few seconds. Although people have done this static stretch before a workout for decades, it is not a good injury-prevention measure. In fact, it may do more harm than good. Because it forces the target muscle to relax, it temporarily makes it weaker. As a result, a strength imbalance can occur between opposing muscle groups. For example, stretching your hamstrings causes them to become significantly weaker than your quadriceps. And that may make you more susceptible to muscle strains, pulls, and tears when you start exercising or playing your sport. What's more, static stretching *reduces* bloodflow to your muscles and decreases the activity of your central nervous system, meaning it inhibits your brain's ability to communicate with your muscles, which limits your capacity to generate force. The bottom line: *Never perform static stretching before you work out or play sports.*

Now, before you abandon static stretching for good, realize that it does have value. That's because improving your "passive" flexibility through static stretches is beneficial in the nonathletic endeavors of everyday life—such as bending, kneeling, and squatting. If you sit behind a computer at work, you'll definitely want to learn a few great static stretches and use them often. But first . . .

THE RULES OF STATIC STRETCHING

When: Any time of day, except before a workout
Why: To improve general flexibility
How: Apply these guidelines:

- Stretch twice a day, every day. Any less frequently and you won't maintain your gains in flexibility—which is why most flexibility plans don't work. Twice a day may seem like a lot, but each "session" will require as little as 4 minutes of your time. Also, there's no need to "warm" your muscles before stretching; that's a myth. So you can stretch at work, while you're watching TV, or while you're cooking dinner.

- Keep in mind that duration matters. You can increase passive flexibility with a static stretch that's held for as little as 5 seconds, but you get optimal gains by holding it between 15 and 30 seconds, the point of diminishing returns.

- Do just one stretch for each tight muscle. Because most of the improvements in flexibility are made on the first stretch, repeating the same movement provides little benefit.

DYNAMIC STRETCHING

A dynamic stretch is the opposite of a static stretch. It's dynamic. It moves. For example: A body-weight lunge is a dynamic stretch for your quadriceps and hips. You quickly move the target muscle in and out of a stretched position. Here's why the difference between static and dynamic stretching matters and why you should do both: Improvements in flexibility are specific to your body position and speed of movement. So if you do only static stretching—as most people are advised—you'll primarily boost your flexibility in that exact posture while moving at a slow speed. While certainly effective if you're a contortionist, it has limited carryover to the flexibility you need in sports and weight training, which require your muscles to stretch at fast speeds in various body positions. That's why dynamic stretching is a necessary component of any program: It improves your "active" flexibility, the kind you need in every type of athletic endeavor.

Walk All Over Plantar Fasciitis

Is the bottom of your foot killing you? You could have plantar fasciitis, a repetitive-stress injury to the connective tissues of the foot. One telltale symptom: The pain sets in when you get out of bed in the morning but subsides as you go about your day. Try thoroughly stretching the calf muscles before a run or rolling a golf ball with the underside of your foot to warm up the ligaments. A tweak to the basic standing calf stretch against a wall—move your back leg inward and point your toes toward the opposite heel—loosens the peroneal muscles of your lower leg, which pull on your foot when they're tight. The tighter they are, the more unevenly your foot will land on the ground, causing inflammation of the plantar fascia. After your run, ice the arch of the foot and take anti-inflammatories. You can also vary the stress by training in different shoes and on different surfaces. If the pain continues, you might need an x-ray to look for a hairline fracture. Remember, pain is the body's way of telling you to stop, so have it checked out before serious damage is done.

Dynamic stretching also excites your central nervous system, and increases bloodflow and strength and power production. So it's the ideal warmup for any activity. And when you regularly perform both dynamic and static stretches, some of the flexibility improvements from one will transfer to the other.

THE RULES OF DYNAMIC STRETCHING

When: As a warmup before any type of workout or sport

Why: To improve performance and reduce injury risk

How: Perform five to eight body-weight exercises or calisthenics at a slow tempo and in a comfortable range of motion. Increase your range and speed with each repetition, until you're performing the movement quickly from start to finish. Do 1 set of 10 repetitions of each exercise, one after the other.

What: Use these movements (shown on the following pages) to stretch your entire body. Do as shown and, for all but number 2, switch sides and repeat the stretch with the opposite arm or leg.

Even More Help for Back Pain

Target your hip flexors. Parking your butt in a chair all day weakens your abs and glutes and shortens your psoas (SO-uhs) muscles. These hip muscles form a girdle that runs from your lower spine across each side of your pelvis and then attaches to the insides of your femurs, explains Bill Hartman, P.T., C.S.C.S.. He recommends the 3-D Psoas Stretch:

3-D PSOAS STRETCH

1ST DIMENSION
With your arms by your sides, step your left foot forward and lower into a lunge with your left knee bent 90 degrees.

2ND DIMENSION
While in the lunge, squeeze your right glute and reach for the sky with your right arm.

3RD DIMENSION
Bend to the left until you feel your right hip stretching. Then twist slightly to the right. Hold for 30 seconds, return to the starting position, switch sides, and repeat. That's 1 set. Do 3 sets, three times a day.

Stretching: More Truth

New research confirms what we've been saying for years: Static stretching doesn't prevent muscle soreness. After examining data from 12 studies, Australian scientists concluded that stretching before, after, or both before and after exercise produces little or no reduction in delayed-onset muscle soreness.

"In the past, stretching was thought to inhibit muscle spasms, allowing the outflow of lactic acid and reducing soreness," says study author Robert Herbert, Ph.D. Now scientists think soreness is probably due to muscle damage, which static stretching won't help, he says. A better way to beat pain: Gradually increase the intensity of any new exercises over a few sessions so your body has time to adjust.

STATIC STRETCHES

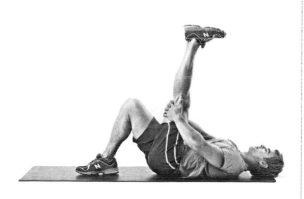

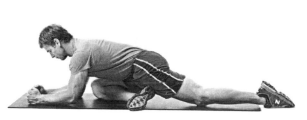

HAMSTRING STRETCH

Lie on your back on the floor. Bend your right knee to 90 degrees, keeping that foot flat on the floor. Raise your left leg as straight as you can with help from your hands clasped around your thigh.
Hold for 30 seconds, then repeat the stretch with your right leg elevated.

BUTT STRETCH

This move stretches the piriformis muscle found deep within the buttocks. A tight piriformis can trigger lower-back pain or irritation of the nearby sciatic nerve. To do the stretch, start by getting on your hands and knees. Bring your right knee forward and move your foot across your body to the outside of your left hip. Slide the other knee back and feel the stretch in the buttocks.
Hold for 30 seconds, then repeat the piriformis stretch with the left leg.

STATIC STRETCHES (continued)

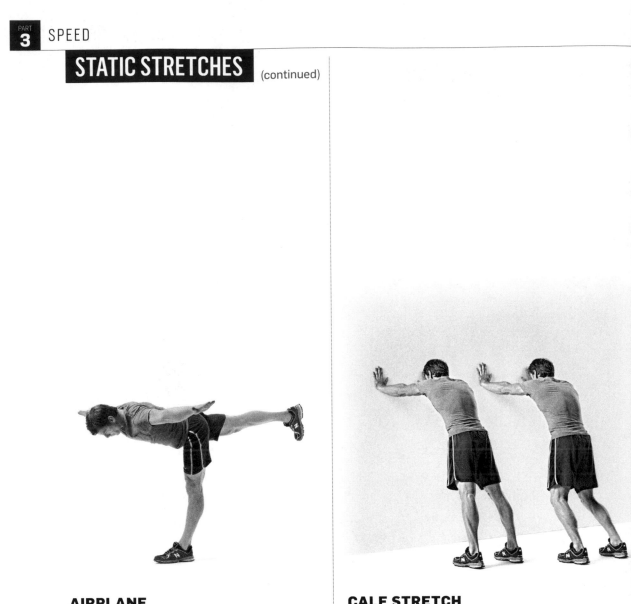

AIRPLANE

Stand with your feet together. Extend your arms out to the sides to form a T. While tightening your abdominal and lower-back muscles, bend forward at the hips, simultaneously raising your right leg off the floor behind you. Try forming a straight line with your back and leg.

Do 5 reps, holding the stretch for 10 seconds each time. Then switch legs and repeat.

CALF STRETCH

Keeping your calves flexible will help you avoid Achilles tendonitis and calf tears. Stand about 3 feet from a wall with your feet about shoulder-width apart. Lean into the wall with your hands against it while keeping your legs straight and your heels on the floor. You'll feel the stretch in the back of your calves.

Hold for 30 seconds, rest, and repeat, this time with your knees slightly bent.

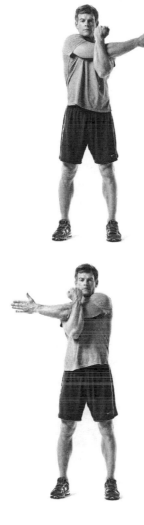

DYNAMIC STRETCHES

Running in place, jumping jacks, and body-weight squats are terrific dynamic stretches. Or you can build a stretching warmup by adding some of these:

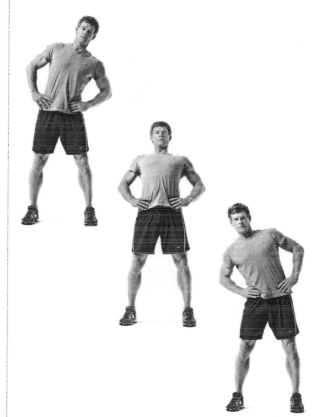

ANTERIOR SHOULDER STRETCH

Move your left arm across the front of your body above your chest. Use your right arm to pull the left arm farther across and into your chest until you feel tension in your deltoid, upper back, and chest.
Hold for 15 seconds, then repeat the stretch with your right arm.

TRUNK ROTATION

Stand with your feet shoulder-width apart and your hands on your hips. Keeping your back straight, bend forward at the hips. Then begin leaning to the right, then rotating around the back, then to your left, and back to the forward position in a smooth, circular motion. Avoid jerky stops at each position. You should keep your hips stable and make circles with your upper body.
Do 5 starting to the right, and then 5 starting to the left.

DYNAMIC STRETCHES

(continued)

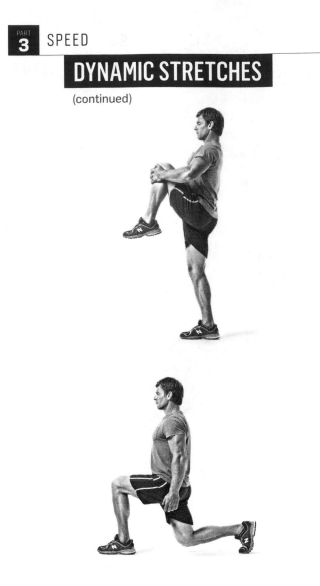

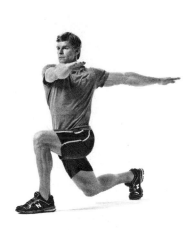

KNEE HUG TO LUNGE

Stand with your feet together. Hug your left knee to your chest. Let go of the knee and step into a lunge. (Be sure to keep your knee aligned above your ankle, never more forward, to avoid injury.) Step back, lifting your knee again. **Do 10 reps, then repeat the lunge with your right leg.**

BACK LUNGE AND TWIST

Start with your feet together. Step back with your right leg and bend your left knee to 90 degrees. Twist your trunk to the left, extending your arms to deepen the stretch. **Do a total of 10 repetitions, then do the back lunge with your left leg.**

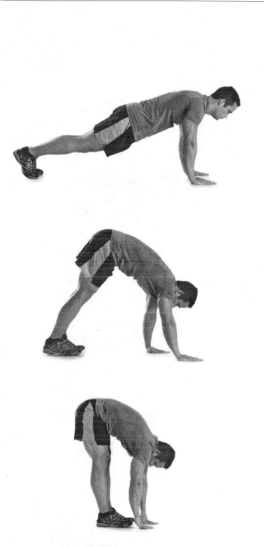

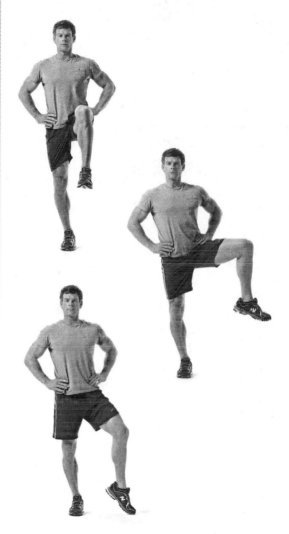

INCHWORM

Start in a pushup position. Slowly walk your feet toward your hands. Your heels can come off the floor, but stop walking forward when the stretch in the backs of your legs starts to feel uncomfortable. Keeping your feet still, slowly walk your arms forward until you are back in the pushup position.
Perform 5 times.

HIP CIRCLE

Stand with your feet together and your hands resting on your hips. Lift your left leg up, bending your knee to 90 degrees. Rotate your hip out to the side and back, then lower the leg. Next raise it back to the side and rotate it forward, then lower.
Do 10 times, then repeat the move with the right leg.

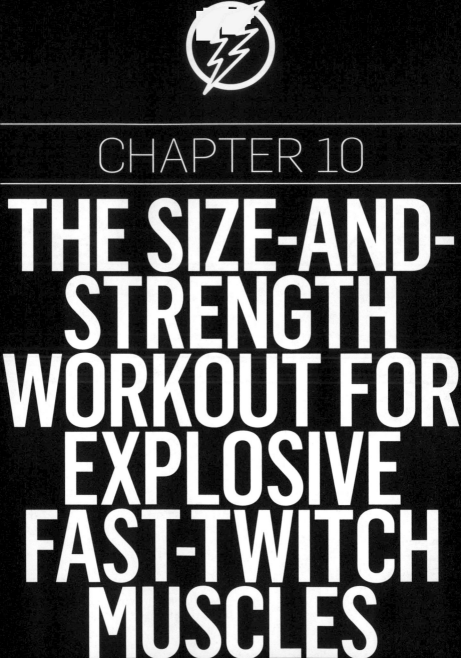

CHAPTER 10

THE SIZE-AND-STRENGTH WORKOUT FOR EXPLOSIVE FAST-TWITCH MUSCLES

In winter, maybe a flat midsection is good enough. But when the shirt comes off in summer, you want a body that looks more like sculpted marble than a blank slate. This workout from Bill Hartman, P.T., C.S.C.S., is based on a system developed for track-and-field athletes by Russian sports scientists and uses a combination of heavy lifting and intense "metabolic accelerators" to fatigue your muscle fibers and turn your body into a work of fine art—in just 4 weeks.

THE SIZE-AND-STRENGTH WORKOUT #1

DIRECTIONS

Alternate between workouts A and B 3 days a week. When two exercises have the same number (3A and 3B, for example), do 1 set of the A exercise and rest for the prescribed time; then do 1 set of the B exercise, and rest again. Repeat until you've completed all sets of each exercise. Then move on to the next pair. End each workout with the accelerator, and then wring out your shirt and go home.

WORKOUT A

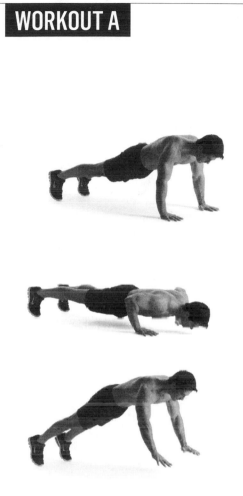

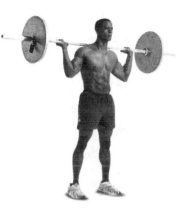

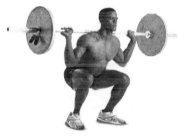

1. EXPLOSIVE PUSHUP

Assume a pushup position. Your body should form a straight line from your head to your ankles. Bend your elbows and lower your body until your chest nearly touches the floor. Then push up with enough force for your hands to come off the floor. Land and repeat.

Week 1: 2 sets of 8 reps
Week 2: 3 sets of 8 reps
Week 3: 2 sets of 10 reps
Week 4: 4 sets of 10 reps
Rest: 90 seconds to 2 minutes between sets

2. BARBELL SQUAT

Hold a barbell across your back using an overhand grip. Keeping your head up and chest high, push your hips back, bend your knees, and lower your body until your thighs are at least parallel to the floor. Push back to the starting position.

Week 1: 2 sets of 4 to 6 reps
Week 2: 3 sets of 3 to 5 reps
Week 3: 2 sets of 2 to 3 reps
Week 4: 3 sets of 2 to 3 reps
Rest: 2 to 3 minutes between sets

WORKOUT A (continued)

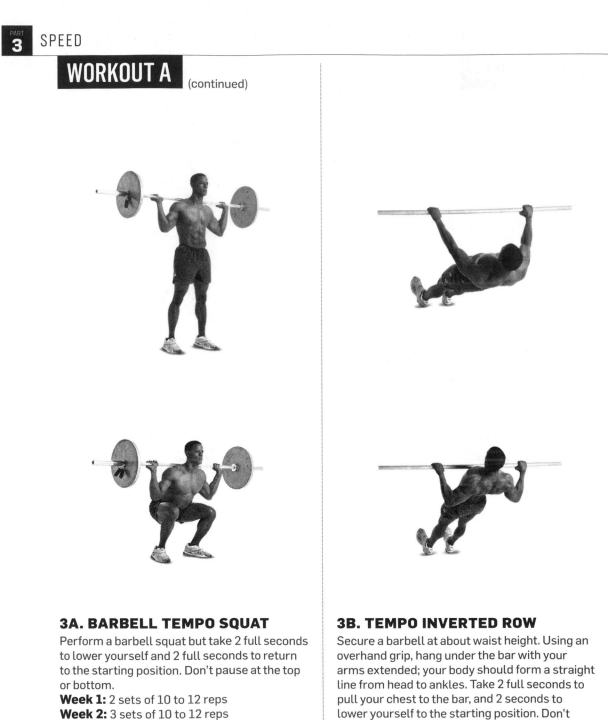

3A. BARBELL TEMPO SQUAT

Perform a barbell squat but take 2 full seconds to lower yourself and 2 full seconds to return to the starting position. Don't pause at the top or bottom.

Week 1: 2 sets of 10 to 12 reps
Week 2: 3 sets of 10 to 12 reps
Week 3: 4 sets of 10 to 12 reps
Week 4: 3 sets of 10 to 12 reps
Rest: 1 minute between sets

3B. TEMPO INVERTED ROW

Secure a barbell at about waist height. Using an overhand grip, hang under the bar with your arms extended; your body should form a straight line from head to ankles. Take 2 full seconds to pull your chest to the bar, and 2 seconds to lower yourself to the starting position. Don't pause at the top or bottom. Use the same sets, reps, and rest as in exercise 3A.

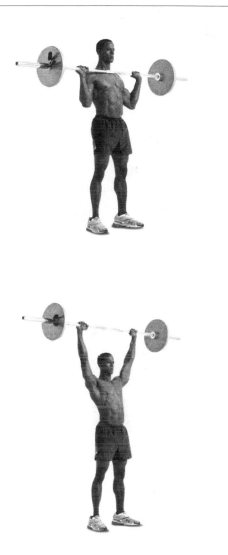

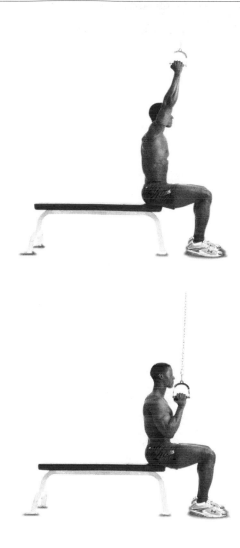

4A. BARBELL SHOULDER PRESS

Grab the bar overhand with your hands just beyond shoulder-width, and hold it in front of your shoulders. Press the bar directly above your head until your arms are straight. Lower and repeat.
Weeks 1 and 2: 2 sets of 12 reps
Weeks 3 and 4: 2 sets of 10 reps
Rest: 1 minute between sets

4B. SINGLE-ARM LAT PULLDOWN

Attach a handle to the high pulley of a cable station. Grab the handle with one hand and sit in front of the weight stack. Without rotating your torso, pull the handle to the side of your chest. Do all your reps, switch hands, and repeat. Use the same sets, reps, and rest as in exercise 4A.

METABOLIC ACCELERATOR

WORKOUT B

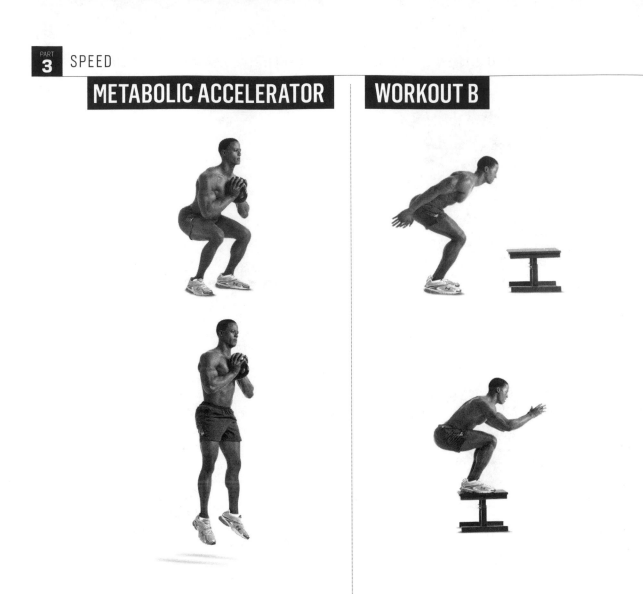

5. KETTLEBELL JUMP

Grab a kettlebell (you can also use a dumbbell) with both hands and hold it against your chest. Squat and jump as many times as you can in 15 seconds. Rest 45 seconds. That's 1 round.
Weeks 1 and 2: 8 rounds
Weeks 3 and 4: 10 rounds

1. BOX JUMP

With your feet shoulder-width apart, dip down and then jump onto a step or box. Step down and repeat. Start with a box that's 18 to 24 inches high, and then use a higher box for weeks 3 and 4.
Week 1: 2 sets of 10 reps
Week 2: 3 sets of 10 reps
Week 3: 2 sets of 8 reps
Week 4: 4 sets of 8 reps
Rest: 90 seconds to 2 minutes between sets

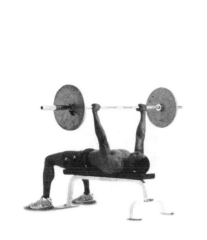

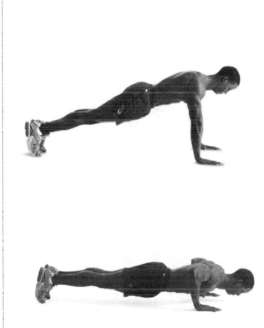

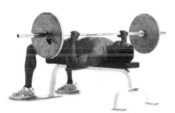

2. BARBELL BENCH PRESS

Grab a barbell and lie on a bench. Using an overhand grip that's just beyond shoulder-width, hold the bar above your sternum, keeping your arms straight. Lower the bar to your chest, and then push it back to the starting position.

Week 1: 2 sets of 4 to 6 reps
Week 2: 3 sets of 3 to 5 reps
Week 3: 2 sets of 2 to 3 reps
Week 4: 4 sets of 2 to 3 reps
Rest: 2 to 3 minutes between sets

3A. TEMPO PUSHUP

Assume a pushup position. Take 2 full seconds to lower yourself to the floor and 2 full seconds to push back up. Don't pause at the top or bottom.

Week 1: 2 sets of 10 to 12 reps
Week 2: 3 sets of 10 to 12 reps
Week 3: 4 sets of 10 to 12 reps
Week 4: 3 sets of 10 to 12 reps
Rest: 1 minute between sets

101

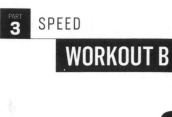

WORKOUT B (continued)

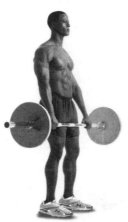

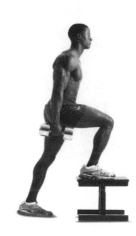

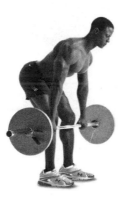

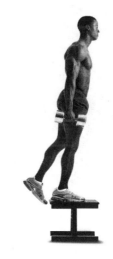

3B. BARBELL STRAIGHT-LEG DEADLIFT

Using an overhand grip, your hands just beyond shoulder-width, grab a bar and hold it at arm's length in front of your thighs. Push your hips back and lower your torso until it's nearly parallel to the floor. Reverse the movement to return to the starting position.

Use the same sets, reps, and rest as in exercise 3A.

4A. DUMBBELL STEPUP

Grab a pair of dumbbells and place your right foot on a box or step. Push through your right heel until your right leg is straight. Lower yourself back down. Do all your reps with your right leg, and repeat with your left.
Weeks 1 and 2: 2 sets of 12 reps
Weeks 3 and 4: 2 sets of 10 reps
Rest: 1 minute between sets

METABOLIC ACCELERATOR

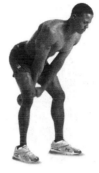

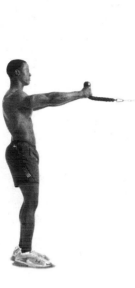

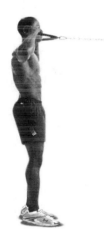

4B. FACE PULL

Attach a rope to the high pulley of a cable station. Grab the ends of the rope with your palms facing each other. Starting with your arms straight, pull the middle of the rope toward your nose (flare your elbows). Pause, and repeat.

Use the same sets, reps, and rest as in exercise 4A.

5. KETTLEBELL SWING

Without rounding your lower back, push your hips back and swing a kettlebell between your legs. Thrust your hips forward and let the weight swing to shoulder level. Start the clock, do 10 swings, and rest; when you hit the 60-second mark, repeat.

Weeks 1 and 2: Go for 8 minutes
Weeks 3 and 4: Go for 10 minutes

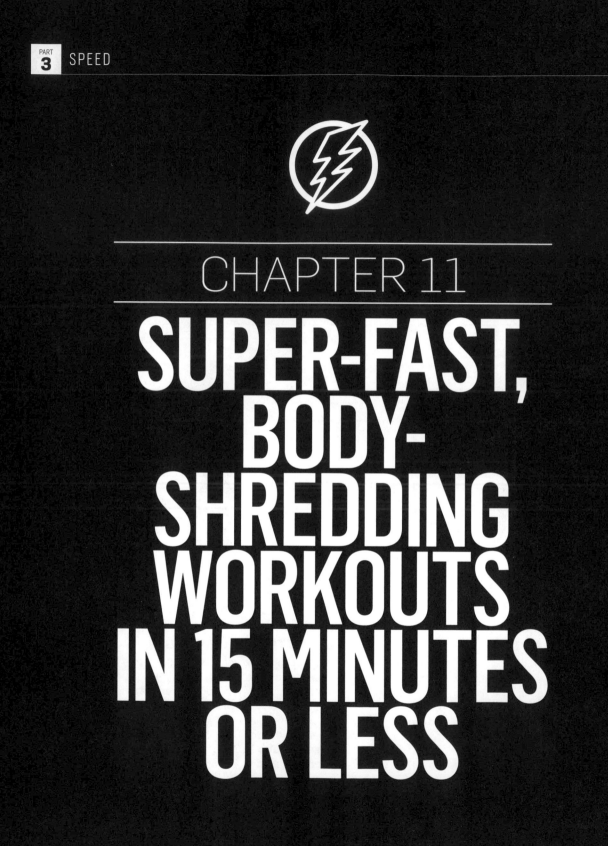

CHAPTER 11

SUPER-FAST, BODY-SHREDDING WORKOUTS IN 15 MINUTES OR LESS

"I DON'T HAVE TIME TO WORK OUT."

Sound familiar? Sure it does. We've all said it at one time or another. Lack of time is the number-one reason men, in survey after survey, give for why they don't exercise.

"Nonsense" is the polite word for this. The more accurate word goes by the initials "B.S."

The fact is, effective, body-altering workouts are like pants: They come in all shapes, sizes, and styles. And lengths. The workouts in this book are all designed to work in a variety of specific time frames, and they work brilliantly. When you have the time to put in a full hour workout, do it. But if you don't? Work out anyway.

Time is no longer an excuse.

If you exercise strategically, with good science on your side, you don't always need an hour. Or even a half hour. When you're up against the clock on a busy day, you can still build the body you want in 15 minutes. According to a recent study published in the *European Journal of Applied Physiology*, 15 minutes of resistance training was just as effective as 35 minutes was in elevating resting energy expenditure for up to 72 hours after the exercise.

That means that you can burn calories and build muscle in half the time you thought possible. And if you're a seriously busy guy, you'll have a much better chance of slimming down with those quick workouts than lengthy gym sessions.

A study in the *International Journal of Sports Medicine* found that volunteers who were trying to lose weight had a much better chance of sticking to an exercise plan if their workouts were cut to 15 minutes.

All of us can find 15 minutes in our day. *Men's Health* magazine has been publishing "15-Minute Workouts" for years, and thousands of men have transformed their bodies as a result.

The following 15-minute workouts are all about building muscle, ripping open your metabolism to unleash its calorie-burning potential, and strengthening your heart, bones, and joints.

You have no more excuses. Pick a workout and make it happen.

15-MINUTE WORKOUT #1

YOUR BODY IS YOUR BARBELL

You'll be surprised how hard you can exercise without a gym with this workout designed by longtime *Men's Health* contributor Craig Ballantyne, M.S., C.S.C.S. These athletic multimuscle moves raise your heart rate, so you incinerate fat while you pack on muscle. As a bonus, they strengthen your core and hone your balance, so you're more injury resistant on the court, slopes, or wherever you play hard.

START HERE

Alternate between the Y Squat and the Spider-Man Pushup for 3 sets of each. Then perform the remaining three exercises as a circuit, one after another (again, without rest). When finished with the Spider-Man Lunge, return to the Squat-Jump Combo and completed the three-exercise circuit twice more.

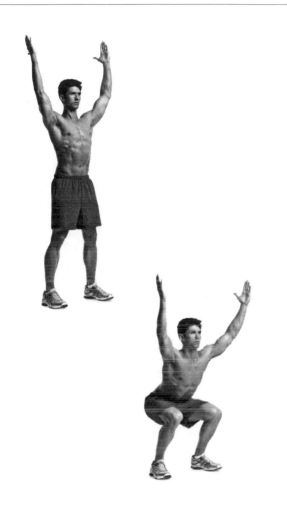

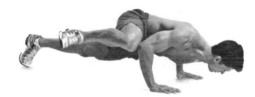

Y SQUAT
Works quads, glutes, and hamstrings.
Stand with your shoulder blades pulled back and your arms extended up and out so your body forms a Y. With your feet slightly more than shoulder-width apart, sit back at your hips to lower your body. Go as low as possible without allowing your back to round. Squeeze your glutes and push yourself back up to the starting position.
Do 12 reps.

SPIDER-MAN PUSHUP
Works chest, arms, and core.
Assume the classic pushup position with your legs straight and your abs tight. As you lower your body, bend your right leg and rotate your right knee outward until it's outside your right elbow. Don't drag your foot, and try not to allow your torso to rotate. As you press yourself up, return the leg to the starting position and repeat, pulling your left knee to your left elbow.
Do 12 to 16 reps, alternating sides.

15-MINUTE WORKOUT #1

(continued)

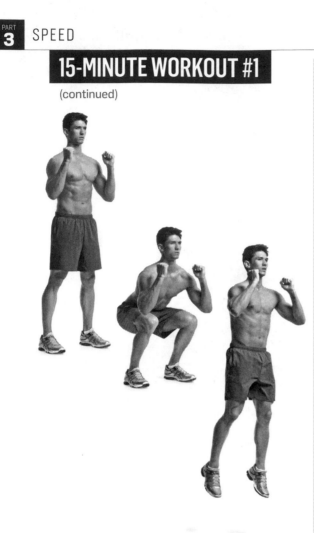

SQUAT + JUMP COMBO
Works fast-twitch muscles in your legs.
Stand with your feet shoulder-width apart. Lower your body as far as you can by pushing your hips back and bending your knees. Pause, and then stand. Squat again, but after this one, jump as high as you can. That's 1 rep. Upon landing, perform a normal squat. Keep alternating between squats and jumps.
Do 8 to 10 reps.

SINGLE-LEG ROMANIAN DEADLIFT
Works lower back, core, and glutes.
Stand on your left foot with your right foot raised behind you, arms hanging down in front of you. Keeping a natural arch in your spine, push your hips back and lower your hands and upper body toward the floor. Squeeze your glutes and press your heel into the floor to return to an upright position. Do all reps, then repeat the exercise while standing on your right foot.
Do 8 to 10 reps per leg.

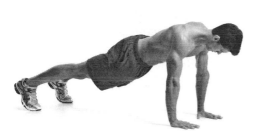

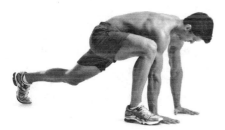

11

Percentage of men who typically stick to just cardio when they're trying to lose weight

SPIDER-MAN LUNGE
Works chest, core, and legs.
Assume the classic pushup position with your hands directly beneath your shoulders, your legs straight, and your abs braced. As you lower yourself to the floor, lift your right foot off the floor, bending your knee, and place the foot outside your right hand. Return to the starting position and lunge forward with your left leg toward your left hand. That's 1 rep.
Do 10 reps.

15-MINUTE WORKOUT #2

THE DUMBBELL BLAST

Most guys have a few sets of dumbbells sitting in the corner that they use for biceps curls and chest presses. But those few exercises barely scratch the surface of the muscle-maximizing potential of these highly versatile hand weights. The following workout builds every single sinew with nothing but a pair (or in some cases just one) of dumbbells.

If you've been reading *Men's Health* magazine for any length of time, you understand our opinion of dumbbells: They're genius. No other single piece of workout equipment is so simple yet so well designed and effective. Dumbbells are the ultimate free weights, allowing you to truly isolate your muscles. Because your dominant side (right hand or left hand) tends to be stronger than the other, when you lift with a straight barbell, you can easily develop muscle imbalances that can lead to injury. Dumbbells eliminate that ability to compensate for weaker muscles. Each side of your body has to work equally hard, creating a balance of power and muscle symmetry.

START HERE

This rapid-fire routine, designed by C. J. Murphy, owner of Total Performance Sports in Everett, Massachusetts, uses just one dumbbell. Do this workout as a circuit; perform each exercise for 45 seconds before moving to the next. After completing one circuit, rest for 1 minute. Then do another one or two circuits. Start with a 15-pound dumbbell. Increase the weight as the workout feels easier, but don't go so heavy that you need to rest between exercises.

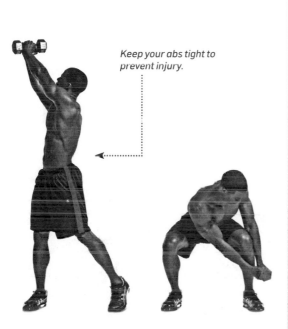

Keep your abs tight to prevent injury.

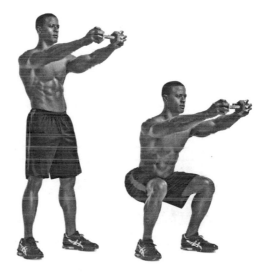

WOODCHOPPER
Works arms, shoulders, and core
Stand with your feet a bit wider than shoulder-width apart. Hold a dumbbell with both hands over your right shoulder, with arms nearly straight. Bend your knees and forcefully rotate your torso left as you draw your arms down and across your body. When your hands go past your left ankle, reverse the motion. Then move the weight over your left shoulder and repeat the move, chopping and rotating right until the weight reaches outside your right ankle.
Do as many reps as you can in 45 seconds, alternating sides.

ARMS-OUT SQUAT
Works quadriceps, hamstrings, shoulders, and back.
Standing with your feet slightly wider than shoulder-width apart, grasp a dumbbell by the ends and hold it straight out from your eyes. Now try to press the ends together as you simultaneously push your hips back, bend your knees, and lower your body until your thighs are parallel to the floor. Pause, and push back up.
Do as many reps as you can in 45 seconds.

15-MINUTE WORKOUT #2

(continued)

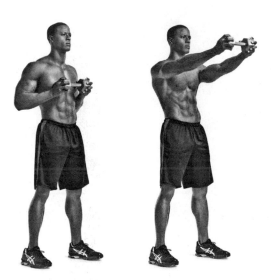

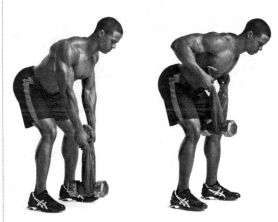

STANDING PRESSOUT
Works shoulders, upper back, and arms.

With your feet shoulder-width apart, hold a dumbbell by its ends and next to your chest. Try to press the ends together as you simultaneously push the dumbbell away from your body and slightly up (to eye level) until your arms are straight. Pause, and pull the dumbbell back as you squeeze your shoulder blades together.
Do as many reps as you can in 45 seconds.

TOWEL ROW
Works shoulders, arms, and chest.

Secure a towel around a dumbbell's handle. Grab an end of the towel with each hand and stand with your feet shoulder-width apart, knees slightly bent. Bend at your hips, keep your lower back flat, and lower your torso until it's almost parallel to the floor. Pull the towel ends to either side of your abdomen. Pause, and lower the towel; repeat without standing back upright.
Do as many reps as you can in 45 seconds.

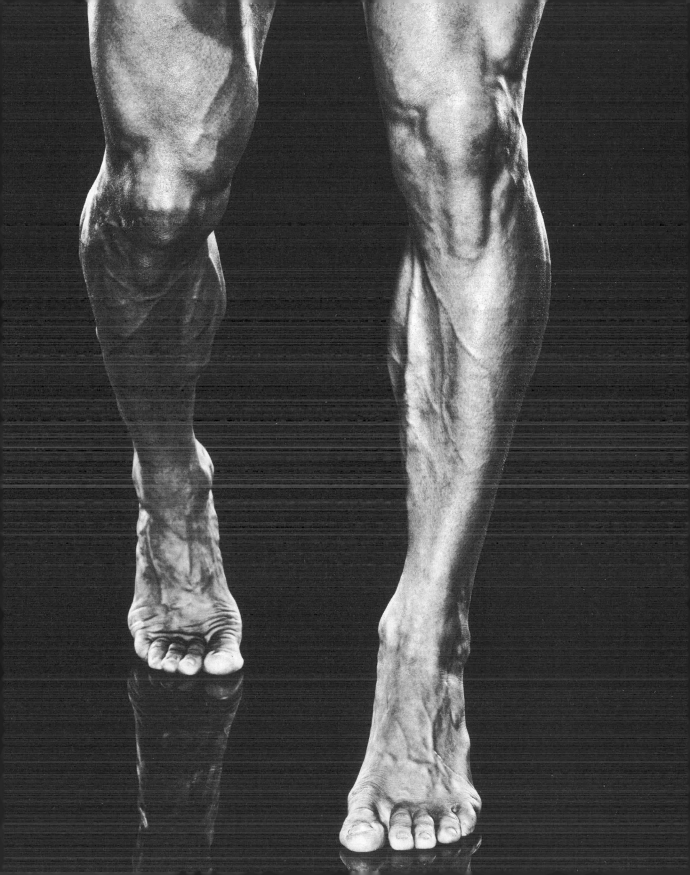

15-MINUTE WORKOUT #3

THE NO-GYM CLASSIC WORKOUTS (ADVANCED)

The workout combines resistance exercises and fat-frying calisthenics for an incredibly effective at-home full-body pump. This is also a terrific "on the road" workout you can do while traveling.

START HERE

Alternate between the Shoulder Press Pushup and the Single-Leg Bench Getup for 3 sets of each. Then perform the remaining four exercises consecutively (again, without rest), doing the circuit three times.

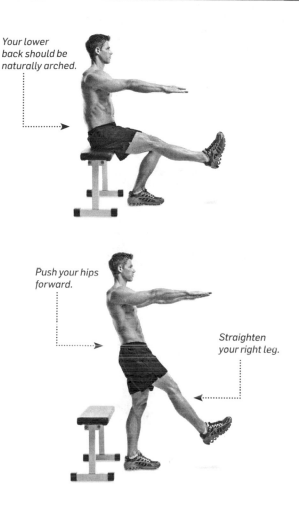

Your lower back should be naturally arched.

Push your hips forward.

Straighten your right leg.

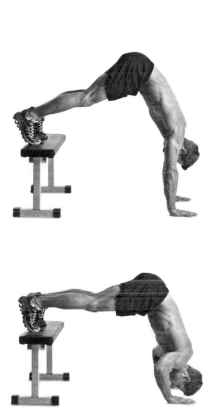

SHOULDER PRESS PUSHUP
Works deltoids, chest, and triceps.
Place your feet on a bench (a bed or chair pushed against a wall can also work) and hands on the floor a foot or two from the bench and slightly wider than shoulder-width apart. Pike your hips up in the air, so you are as vertical as can be. Slowly bend your arms to lower your head to the floor. Pause, and push with your shoulders and triceps back to the start position.
Do 10 reps.

SINGLE-LEG BENCH GETUP
Works quadriceps and calves.
Sit on a bench (or bed or chair) with your back upright and hold your arms straight out in front of your body at shoulder height, parallel to the floor. Raise your left foot off the floor. Without leaning forward, press your body to a standing position. (If this is too difficult, try sliding your foot slightly back toward your body in the starting position.) Sit back down and repeat.
Do 4 to 6 reps with each leg.

15-MINUTE WORKOUT #3
(continued)

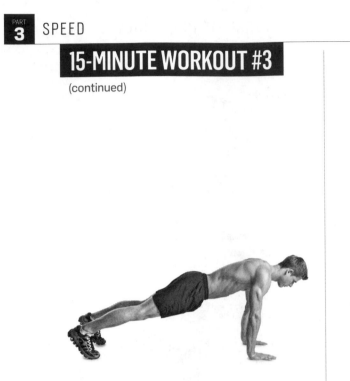

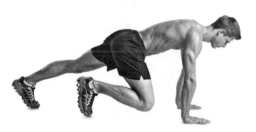

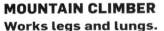

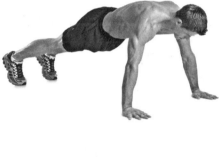

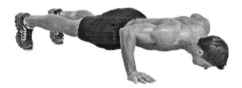

MOUNTAIN CLIMBER
Works legs and lungs.
Assume the classic pushup position with your hands on the floor directly under your shoulders. Brace your abs and straighten your legs behind you. This is the starting position. Lift one foot off the floor and bring your knee toward your chest. Straighten your leg back out, move your other knee to your chest, and return that leg to the starting position. Alternate right, left, right, left as fast as you can with good form.
Do 10 reps per leg.

WIDE-GRIP PUSHUP
Works chest and arms.
Assume the classic pushup position with your legs straight and your abs tight. Place your hands on the floor wider than shoulder-width apart. Bend your elbows and lower your chest toward the floor until your upper arms are parallel with the floor. Press back to the starting position.
Do 20 reps.

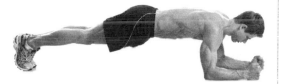

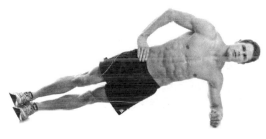

PLANK
Works core.
Get into the pushup position, but bend your elbows and rest your weight on your forearms. Your body should form a straight line from your shoulders to your ankles. Brace your core and hold.
Reps: Hold for 1 minute.

SIDE PLANK
Works core.
Lie on your side and use your forearm to support your body. Raise your hips until your body forms a straight line from shoulder to ankles. Hold and repeat for the other side.
Reps: Hold for 1 minute per side.

15-MINUTE WORKOUT #4

THE MUSCLE DEFINER

If you want to build muscles that pop, you need to lift with high intensity and heavy weights, says veteran strength coach Mark Philippi. The power exercises in the following workout target your fast-twitch muscles, the ones with the greatest potential for size and strength. You'll be using heavy weight. Try to perform each movement quickly while maintaining control of the weight at all times.

START HERE

Do this circuit three times, adding a little more weight each time. Rest 30 seconds between circuits.

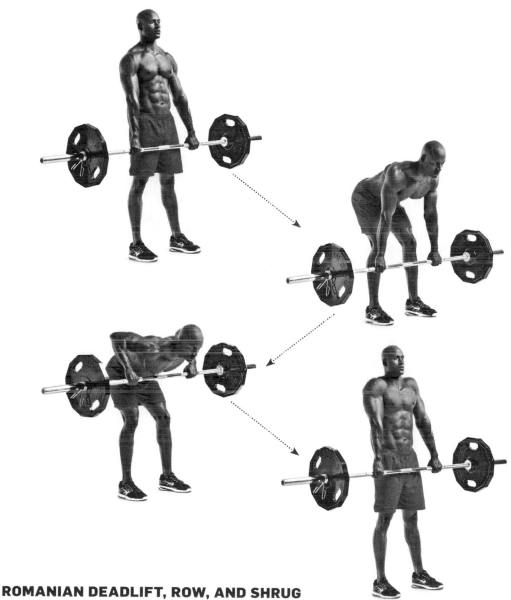

ROMANIAN DEADLIFT, ROW, AND SHRUG
Works total body.
Stand with your feet shoulder-width apart and knees slightly bent. Using an overhand grip (hands about shoulder-width apart), hold a barbell in front of your thighs. Push your hips backward and lower the bar below your knees. Bend at the hips. When your back is flat and parallel to the floor, pull the bar up to your sternum and lower it. Stand up, keeping the bar as close to your body as possible. Shrug your shoulders. That's 1 rep.
Do 5 reps.

15-MINUTE WORKOUT #4

(continued)

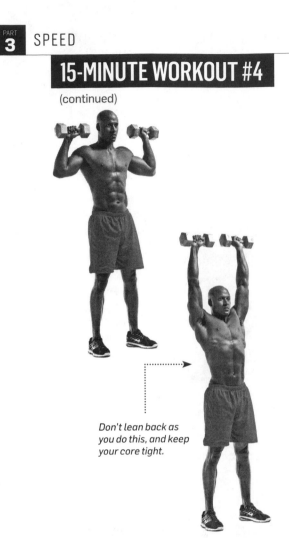

*Don't lean back as
you do this, and keep
your core tight.*

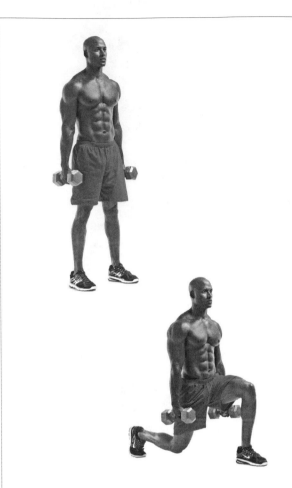

DUMBBELL STANDING PRESS
Works arms and shoulders.
Hold a pair of dumbbells at shoulder level,
palms facing forward. Press the weights
straight overhead, and then lower them.
Do 8 reps.

DUMBBELL LUNGE
Works legs, hips, and glutes.
Stand holding dumbbells at your sides, palms
facing inward. Step forward with your right foot
and lower your body until your front and back
knees are bent 90 degrees and your back knee
is about an inch off the floor. Push back up and
repeat with the other leg. That's 1 rep.
Do 4 lunges with each leg.

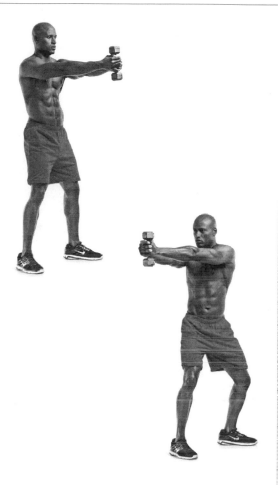

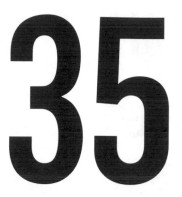

35

Percentage of men who believe they need to train at least 5 days a week in order to see their abs

DUMBBELL ROTATION
Works arms and core.
Hold a dumbbell vertically with both hands. Raise it until your arms are parallel with the floor, and rotate it to just past one shoulder (without moving your lower body). Return.
Do 15 reps per side.

15-MINUTE WORKOUT #5

THE CLASSIC POWER LIFTER WORKOUT

You don't need much time to build great power. In fact, you need only three moves to train every major muscle and move thousands of pounds in a single workout. Power lifters focus on these training classics—the barbell squat, bench press, and deadlift—because, when done right, they are so effective and efficient. The key is using heavy weight and pushing yourself on each lift, says Mike Robertson, M.S., C.S.C.S., a strength coach in Indianapolis.

START HERE

Begin by doing 2 light sets of barbell squats (10 to 12 reps), resting for 90 seconds in between. Next, load the bar with a weight you can lift only six times with your best effort. Perform 5 flawless repetitions, then rest for 2 minutes before moving on. Do the same for the other two exercises.

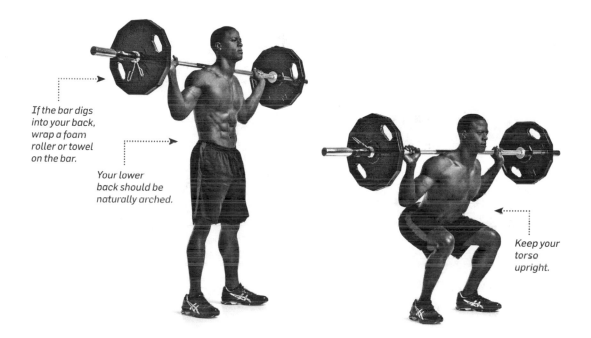

If the bar digs into your back, wrap a foam roller or towel on the bar.

Your lower back should be naturally arched.

Keep your torso upright.

BARBELL SQUAT
Works quadriceps, glutes, and calves.
Stand with your feet hip-width apart, and hold the barbell across the back of your shoulders with an overhand grip. With your back naturally arched, bend at the hips and knees until your thighs are at least parallel to the floor. Then return to a standing position.
Do 2 light sets of 10 to 12 reps, then a heavy set of 5.

15-MINUTE WORKOUT #5 (continued)

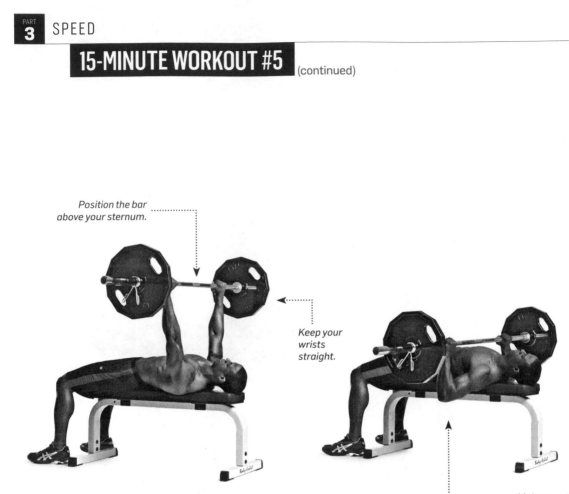

Position the bar above your sternum.

Keep your wrists straight.

Make sure the bar is directly above your elbows throughout the exercise.

BARBELL BENCH PRESS
Works chest, front deltoids, and triceps.

Lie on a bench with your feet flat on the floor. Grab the bar with your hands more than shoulder-width apart, and hold it over your chest. Squeeze your shoulder blades down and together. As you lower the weight to your chest, pull your elbows toward your sides. Pause, then push the weight back up while by driving your head and upper body into the bench.
Do 2 light sets of 10 to 12 reps, then a heavy set of 5.

For safety, keep the bar as close to your body as possible when lifting.

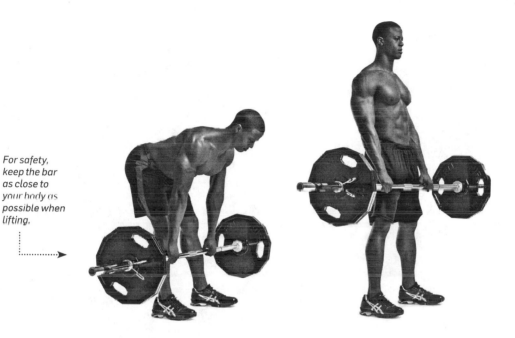

BARBELL DEADLIFT
Works glutes, hamstrings, core, shoulders, hips, and back.

Stand with a bar on the floor in front of you so it just touches your shins. Push your hips back and grasp the bar with your hands just outside your calves with an overhand grip. Keeping your back straight and chest up, drive your heels into the floor and stand up, raising the weight. Then lower the bar back to the floor.

Do 2 light sets of 10 to 12 reps, then a heavy set of 5.

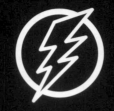

CHAPTER 12

FOUR WEEKS TO A BEACH BODY

If you want to look like an athlete, train like an athlete. Some of the world's best-conditioned men use this workout, but it was designed with you in mind. As a collegiate strength and conditioning coach, Robert dos Remedios, M.A., C.S.C.S., works with guys of average strength and size every day. His job is to turn them into elite performers.

By developing explosive speed, strength, and power, these men also attain something more—the chiseled look of a high-performance athlete. Use this plan to redefine your body and raise your game. The training is short, intense, and if you put in the effort, highly effective.

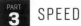
THE EXERCISES

DIRECTIONS

Perform this workout three times a week with at least a day of rest between sessions. Do each exercise in the order shown. Complete 3 or 4 sets of each exercise except for the final movement (Plank with Weight Transfer), which you perform just once for 30 to 60 seconds. Use this schedule for reps and rest.

WEEK 1

• Perform 5 reps of the first exercise (Clean Pull) and rest 90 to 120 seconds between sets.

• Do 10 reps for exercises 2 through 7, resting 60 seconds between sets.

• Do the Plank with Weight Transfer (page 132) once for 30 to 60 seconds.

WEEK 2

• Perform 3 reps of the first exercise (Clean Pull) and rest 90 to 120 seconds between sets.

• Do 5 reps for exercises 2 through 7, resting 90 seconds between sets.

• Do the Plank with Weight Transfer (page 132) once for 30 to 60 seconds.

WEEK 3

• Perform 5 reps of the first exercise (Clean Pull) and rest 90 to 120 seconds between sets.

• Do 8 reps for exercises 2 through 7, resting 60 seconds between sets.

• Do the Plank with Weight Transfer (page 132) once for 30 to 60 seconds.

WEEK 4

• Perform 2 reps of the first exercise (Clean Pull) and rest 90 to 120 seconds between sets.

• Do 3 reps for exercises 2 through 7, resting 90 seconds between sets.

• Do the Plank with Weight Transfer (page 132) once for 30 to 60 seconds.

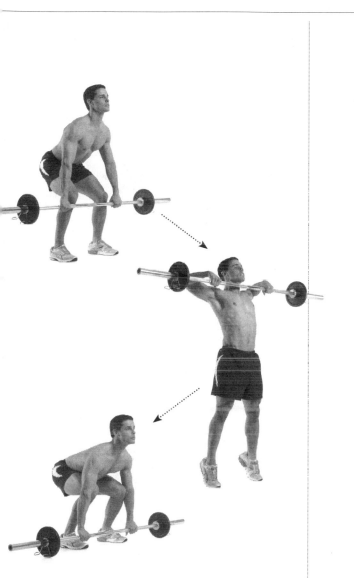

CLEAN PULL

Load a barbell and roll it to your shins. Squat down and grab the bar overhand (palms facing you). In one explosive motion, pull the bar off the floor, straighten your legs, rise onto your toes, and shrug your shoulders. Then lower the bar to the floor.

Keep your arms straight as you shrug your shoulders.

FRONT STEPUP

Stand in front of a bench holding a barbell across the front of your shoulders. Place your right foot on the bench and push your body up until you're standing on the bench. Complete your reps on one leg before switching to the other leg and repeating.

Keep your elbows high and upper arms parallel to the floor.

129

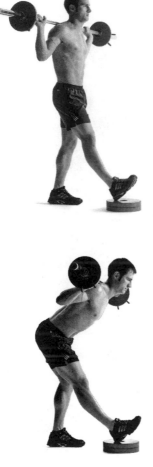

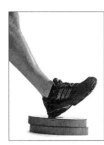

SPLIT GOOD MORNING

Stand holding a barbell across the back of your shoulders. Place one heel on two weight plates just in front of you. With that leg straight and your back leg slightly bent, bend forward. Return to the starting position. Do all your reps before switching sides.

Bend forward as far as possible without rounding your back.

PUSH JERK

Stand holding a barbell in front of your shoulders. Dip slightly, and then in one motion straighten your legs and push the weight overhead. When your arms are almost fully extended, widen your base and bend your knees. Return to the starting position.

Hold the bar with an overhand grip (palms forward).

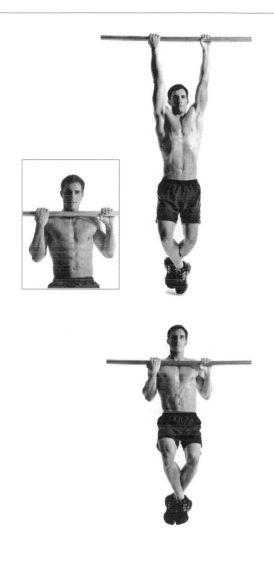

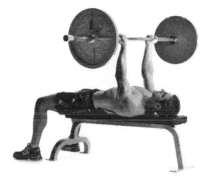

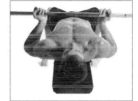

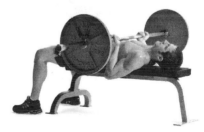

MIXED-GRIP PULLUP

Grab a pullup bar with a mixed grip (one palm facing toward you, the other facing away). Hang with your arms straight and brace your abs. Pull yourself up until your chin is over the bar. Then slowly lower yourself. Reverse your grips on the next set.

Space your hands about shoulder-width apart.

REVERSE-GRIP BENCH PRESS

Lie flat on a bench. Grab the barbell using an underhand grip (palms up) and hold it over your chest with straight arms. Pull your shoulder blades back and down. Lower the bar to the center of your chest. Then push the bar back up.

Pull your elbows toward your body as you lower the bar.

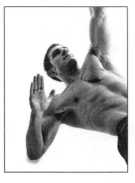

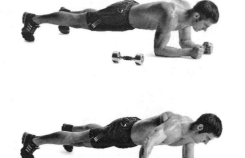

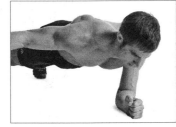

ONE-ARM HORIZONTAL PULLUP

Lie under a secure waist-high bar with your
heels on the floor and grab the bar with one
arm extended over the center of your body.
Pull up toward the bar, lower yourself, and
repeat with the other arm. Too hard? Bend your
knees or use two hands.

Reach your free arm up toward the ceiling,
as if punching up.

PLANK WITH WEIGHT TRANSFER

Assume the plank position with a light weight
to the outside of your right elbow. Pick up the
weight with your right hand and pass it to your
left hand. Place the weight to your left. Move
the weight back to the other side. Continue for
30 to 60 seconds.

Brace your abs to keep your torso from
rotating as you lift the weight.

YOU THINK YOU'RE GOOD?

PONDER THESE HUMBLING NUMBERS

3,416
Most pushups ever performed in 1 hour

3,989
Most parallel-bar dips done in 1 hour

445
Most chinups done in 1 hour

1,005
Heaviest weight, in pounds, lifted in the bench press

1,200
Heaviest weight, in pounds, lifted in the barbell squat

1,003
Heaviest weight, in pounds, lifted in the deadlift

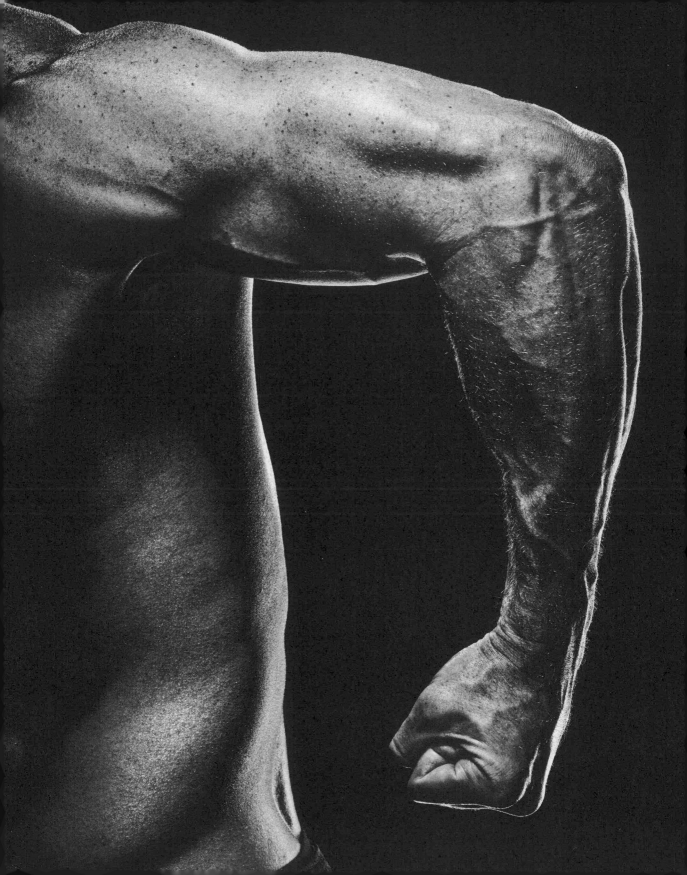

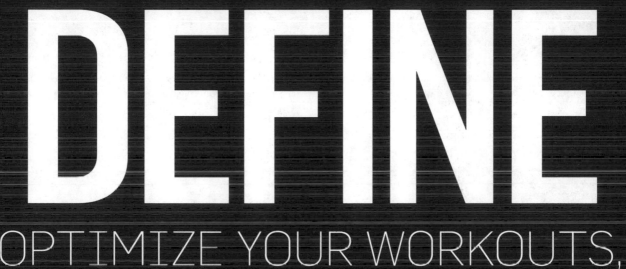

PART FOUR

DEFINE

OPTIMIZE YOUR WORKOUTS,
STRIP AWAY FAT, AND
LEAVE NO MUSCLE BEHIND

CHAPTER 13

25 WAYS TO BUILD BIGGER BICEPS

F

or decades, the dumbbell curl has been helping us build bigger biceps—but it's also stripped us of our imagination. After all, how often do you try a new variation of this classic arm exercise? If it's not every 4 weeks, then you need to shake up your workout to achieve faster results. Start today with this simple guide. By mixing and matching any of the five hand positions and five body positions described on the next few pages, you can instantly create 25 different versions of the curl. The upshot: You'll never run out of new ways to build your biceps.

THE RIGHT WAY TO CURL

CHOOSE YOUR HAND POSITION

Let the dumbbells hang at arm's length straight down from your shoulders. Then, without moving your upper arms, bend your elbows and curl the dumbbells as close to your shoulders as you can. Pause, and slowly lower the weights back to the starting position. Each time you return to the start, straighten your arms completely.

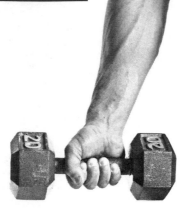

STANDARD
With your palms facing forward, grip the handles in the middle.
The benefit: This is the hand position for the classic dumbbell curl, which targets your biceps brachii, the largest muscle on the front of your upper arm.

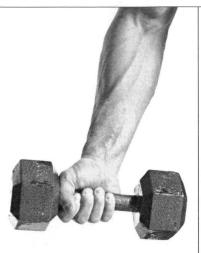

THUMB OFFSET
With your palms facing forward, touch the outside heads of the dumbbells with your thumbs.
The benefit: As you curl the weight, you're forcing your biceps brachii to work harder to keep your forearm rotated outward (so your palms are up).

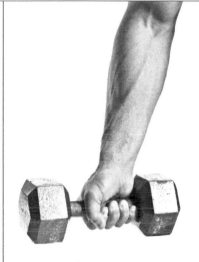

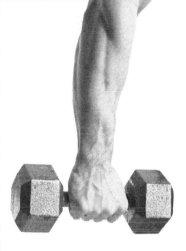

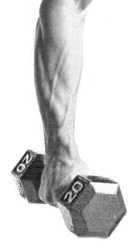

PINKY OFFSET

With your palms facing forward, touch the inside heads of the dumbbells with your pinky fingers.
The benefit: This tweak shifts the way the weight is distributed, providing more variety to keep your muscles growing.

REVERSE

Turn your arms so your palms face behind you.
The benefit: You'll really feel it in your forearms: This position targets your brachioradialis, but it decreases the activity of your biceps brachii.

HAMMER

Keep your palms facing each other.
The benefit: You're forcing your brachialis muscle to work harder for the entire movement. Building your brachialis can make your arms look thicker.

CHOOSE YOUR BODY POSITION

Lifting the weight is only part of the story. There are several ways to perform a curl that each offer a different benefit. Try 'em all!

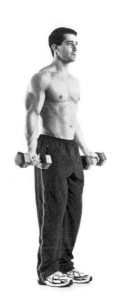

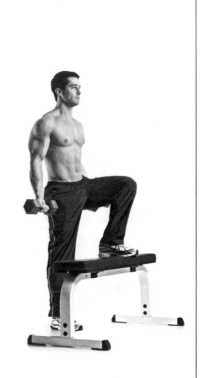

STANDING
Stand tall with your feet shoulder-width apart. **The benefit:** More muscle. Any time you're standing, you engage more core muscles than when you sit.

SPLIT STANCE
Stand tall and place one foot in front of you on a bench or step that's just higher than knee level. **The benefit:** Stronger abs. This stance forces your hip and core muscles to work harder in order to keep your body stable.

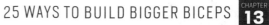

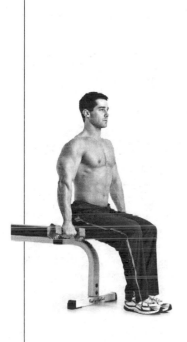

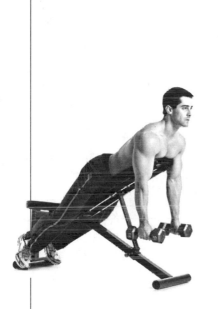

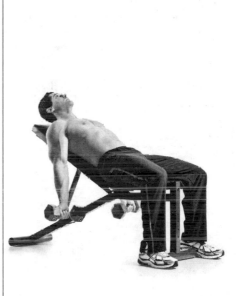

SEATED

Sit tall on a bench
or Swiss ball.
The benefit: Better form.
Performing the exercise
while seated may make you
less likely to rock your torso
back and forth ("cheat")
as you curl the weight.

DECLINE

Lie chest down on a bench
set at 45 degrees.
The benefit: Thicker arms.
Lying on a decline causes
your arms to hang in front
of your body, a position
that challenges your
brachialis more.

INCLINE

Lie on your back on
a bench set at 45 degrees.
The benefit: Bigger
guns. Lying on an incline
causes your arms to hang
behind your body, which
emphasizes the long head
of your biceps brachii to
a greater degree.

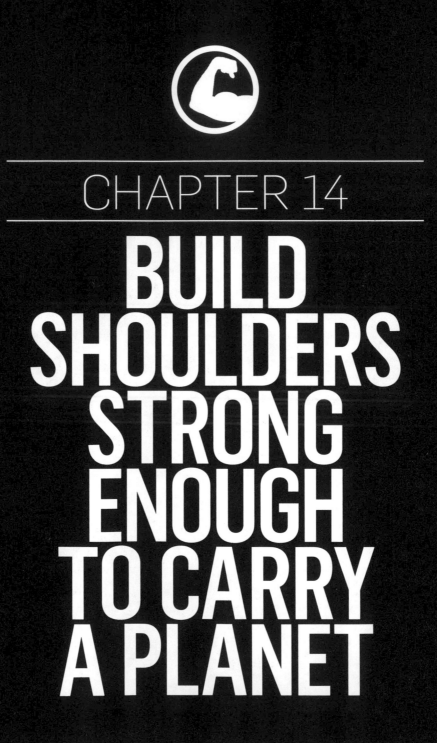

CHAPTER 14

BUILD SHOULDERS STRONG ENOUGH TO CARRY A PLANET

A

tlas shrugged. You have to lift. Sure, most days it feels like you're carrying around a planet or two. But building strong yet supple shoulders is one of the biggest keys to overall fitness. Why? Think about it: Virtually every athletic movement you can think of involves the shoulders. So don't skimp. The workout in this chapter is comprehensive and designed to build strength, of course, but also to keep your shoulder joints healthy and flexible.

THE WORKOUT

The best way to build muscle isn't always the most obvious. For instance, conventional wisdom says that if your shoulders are weak, you're not working them hard enough. But in fact just the opposite is true, especially when it comes to the most obvious exercise. "Men do entirely too many shoulder presses," says Jon Crosby, C.S.C.S., performance director for Velocity Sports Performance. "Excessive pressing exercises can destabilize your shoulders by overworking the front portions of the muscles, which eventually causes the shoulder joints to be pulled out of alignment." So instead of growing stronger, your shoulders—and all the muscles that attach to the shoulder joints, including those of your chest and arms—become weaker over time.

The solution is this 4-week plan, courtesy of Crosby. It's designed to work the entire shoulder girdle—all the muscles that hold your upper-arm bone in its socket and allow the shoulder blade to move. And although logic might suggest that such a well-rounded approach would require extra time in the gym, Crosby took into account that most chest and back exercises involve your shoulders—so you need to use this workout only once a week. Perform workout A in the first 2 weeks and workout B in weeks 3 and 4. Do the exercises in the order shown, finishing all sets of an exercise before moving on to the next one.

THE PAYOFF

Greater strength. The alternating shoulder press in this workout helps you look great all over. Because you work each arm separately, both sides of your body are trained evenly—helping you avoid muscle imbalances.

A bulletproof upper body. This workout emphasizes your rotator cuffs—the primary stabilizers of the shoulder joints. Since the shoulders are the most unstable joints in the body, shoring them up helps protect you from injury and allows you to lift more in every upper-body exercise.

The ultimate pump. This routine incorporates a sequence called the Javorek complex, named after former Romanian Olympic weight-lifting coach Istvan Javorek. It works your shoulders from five angles, forcing a surge of blood that'll make your upper body appear larger right after your workout.

How Strong Are Your Shoulders?

The classic military press builds the largest muscles of your shoulders, including your deltoids, rotator cuffs, and trapezius, making it a great exercise to measure shoulder strength.

Sit on a bench with your feet flat on the floor and grab an empty bar with your hands slightly more than shoulder-width apart. (Use a spotter.) Keeping your back straight, press the bar overhead until your arms are straight, then lower it to the top of your chest. Do 10 repetitions, rest 60 seconds, then add 10 to 20 pounds and repeat for a set of 8 repetitions. Rest again, add another 10 pounds, and do a third set, this time of 5 repetitions. Continue adding weight in increments of 5 to 10 pounds—increase your rests to 2 to 3 minutes—until you work up to the heaviest weight you can lift five times. That's your 5-repetition maximum, or 5-rep max.

TRACK YOUR PROGRESS
Record your 5-rep max in the chart here. Then follow the workout in this chapter and retest yourself every 2 weeks.

Start	[Weight in Pounds]
Week 2	[Weight in Pounds]
Finish	[Weight in Pounds]

WORKOUT A: WEEKS 1 & 2

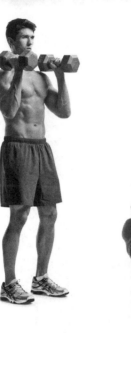

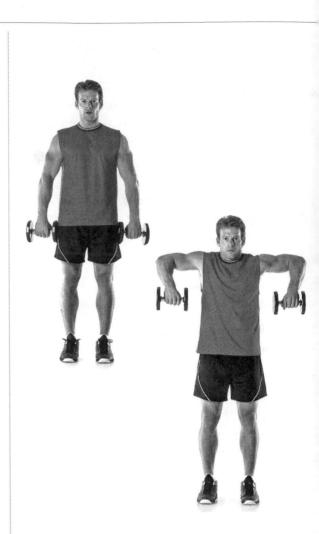

ALTERNATING SHOULDER PRESS

Stand holding a dumbbell in each hand just above your shoulders, with a neutral grip (palms facing each other). Press the weight in your right hand straight above you until your arm is fully extended, then slowly lower the weight to the starting position. Now press the dumbbell in your left hand straight up and lower it. Continue to alternate arms throughout the set.
In week 1, do 2 sets of 10 repetitions with each arm; in week 2, do 3 sets of 8 reps with each arm. Rest for 60 to 90 seconds between sets.

DUMBBELL UPRIGHT ROW (WIDE)

Stand holding a pair of dumbbells at arm's length at your sides, your palms facing behind you. Keeping your forearms pointed down, lift your upper arms until they are parallel with your shoulders then slowly lower them.
Perform 2 sets of 10 repetitions in week 1, and 3 sets of 8 reps in week 2. Rest for 60 to 90 seconds between sets.

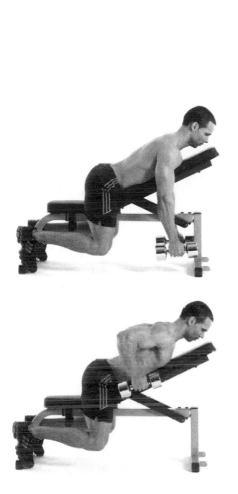

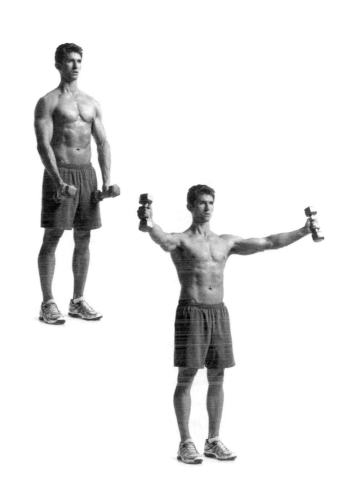

INCLINE ROW

Lie facedown on a bench that's set at a
45-degree incline, and hold a light dumbbell in
each hand. Your arms should hang straight
down. Keeping your head down, pull the
weights up until your upper arms are parallel
to the floor. Squeeze your shoulder blades
together. Pause, then reverse the movement to
return to the starting position.
**Perform 2 sets of 12 repetitions, resting for
45 to 60 seconds between sets.**

STANDING SCAPTION

Stand holding a light pair of dumbbells in front
of your thighs with a neutral grip (your palms
facing each other). Raise your arms forward
and out at 45-degree angles until they're at eye
level. The weights should point to 10 o'clock
and 2 o'clock at the top of the move. Slowly
lower your arms.
**Perform 2 sets of 12 repetitions, resting for
45 to 60 seconds between sets.**

WORKOUT B: WEEKS 3 & 4

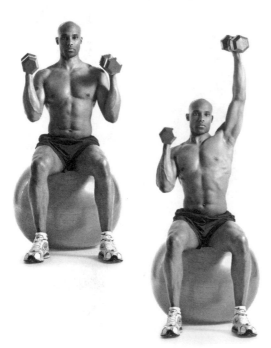

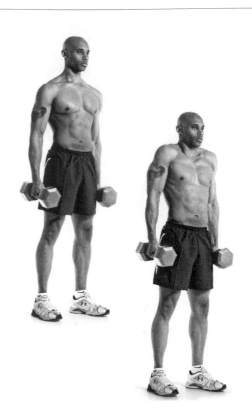

SWISS-BALL ALTERNATING SHOULDER PRESS

Sit on a Swiss ball with your feet flat on the floor. Hold a pair of dumbbells just above your shoulders with a neutral grip, your palms facing each other. Press the weights overhead until your arms are straight. Keeping your right arm extended, slowly lower the weight in your left hand to its starting position, then press it back up. Next, keeping your left arm extended, lower the weight in your right hand and press it back up. Continue alternating arms.
Perform 3 sets of 6 repetitions with each arm, resting for 60 to 90 seconds between sets.

DUMBBELL SHRUG

Stand holding a heavy dumbbell in each hand at arm's length, with your palms facing the sides of your thighs. Keeping your arms straight, shrug your shoulders up as if you were trying to touch them to your ears. Pause, then slowly lower your shoulders until your arms hang down as far as possible.
Do 3 sets of 8 repetitions in week 3, and 4 sets of 5 reps in week 4. Rest for 60 to 90 seconds between sets.

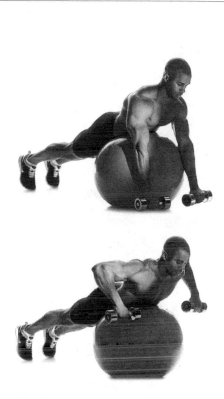

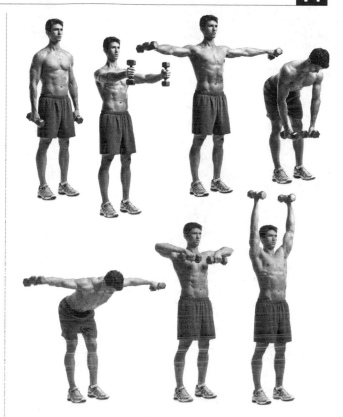

LYING SWISS-BALL ROW TO EXTERNAL ROTATION

Holding a light dumbbell in each hand, lie facedown on a Swiss ball with your chest off the ball so your body is inclined. Your arms should hang down in front of the ball, palms facing your feet. Keeping your neck straight, slowly pull the weights up until your upper arms are parallel to the floor, then rotate your forearms forward until your palms face the floor. Pause, then reverse the motion to lower the weights to the starting position.
Perform 2 sets of 10 repetitions, resting for 45 to 60 seconds between sets.

JAVOREK COMPLEX

Stand holding a pair of dumbbells, arms at your sides, palms facing each other. Raise your arms in front of you until they're parallel to the floor. Lower the weights and repeat for a total of 6 reps. Now raise your arms out from your sides until they're parallel to the floor, and lower them. Again, complete 6 reps. Next, bend forward at the waist until your torso is almost parallel to the floor. Raise your arms out to your sides, lower them, and repeat for a total of 6 reps. Stand up and place your hands in front of your thighs, palms toward you. Pull both weights up until they're just below your chin. Lower and repeat for 6 reps. Finally, turn your palms so they face each other, curl the weights up to your shoulders, and press them overhead. Reverse the move and repeat for 6 reps.
Perform 2 sets, resting for 90 seconds between sets.

BONUS CHAPTER

MASTER
THE PULLUP

Guys avoid pullups for mostly one reason: They're hard. And if you can't do even one, it's embarrassing to just hang there. Memories of seventh-grade gym class, matchstick arms, and laughing classmates aren't easily forgotten.

But if you can't complete at least 10 in a row with perfect form, or haven't boosted your total by three or four in the past year, you're missing out. The pullup is the best way to work the biggest muscle group in your upper body: your latissimus dorsi. If you're not improving, they're not growing.

The solution? Use our custom guide to crossing the bar. Because the pullup is a body-weight exercise, it requires a different approach than the bench press and arm curl. Instead of adjusting the amount of weight you lift to match your workout—as you would with free-weight or machine exercises— you'll adjust your workout based on your ability. So the number of pullups you can do will dictate the routine you follow. This ensures that you're always using the right pullup plan for you—whether you can already pump out double digits or can't yet manage a single one.

The result: You'll have a better body—and the ghosts of junior high will finally be laid to rest.

TEST YOUR LIMIT

Before you get started, determine how many pullups you can do.

Here's the drill: Hang from a pullup bar using an overhand grip that's just beyond shoulder-width apart, your arms completely straight. Cross your feet behind you. Without moving your lower body, pull yourself as high as you can; your chin should rise above the bar. Pause momentarily, then lower your body until your arms are straight, and repeat.

Record your total, then find the pullup routine below that corresponds to your best effort. Do that workout twice a week, resting at least 2 days between sessions.

After 4 weeks, retest yourself. Depending on your score, either advance to the next workout or repeat the same routine for another 4 weeks.

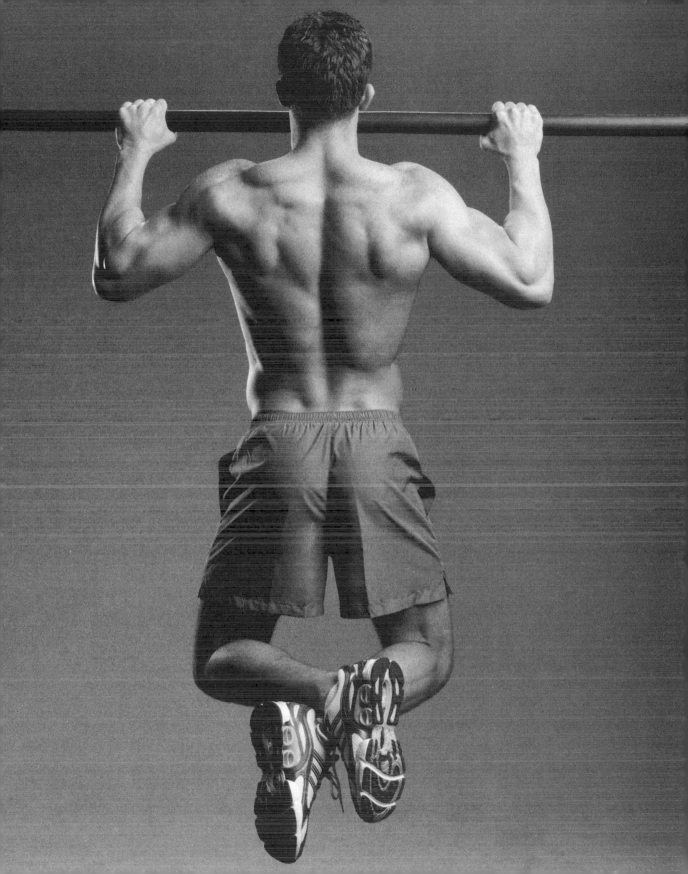

YOUR BEST EFFORT: 0 TO 1

The problem: You're not strong enough to lift your body weight.

The fix: Turn your weakness into an advantage with heavy "negatives." Doing only the lowering portion of an exercise with a heavier weight than you can lift is a fast way to build strength.

How to do it: First, a couple of definitions.

- **Chinup:** This is the same movement as a pullup, but you'll use a shoulder-width, underhand grip. Because your biceps are more involved, it's a little easier than the pullup.

- **Neutral-grip pullup:** Again, it's the same basic movement, but you'll grip the parallel bars of the pullup station so your palms are facing each other. This is harder than a chinup, but not as hard as a pullup.

Now follow the workout schedule below, using this method of performing negatives:

Place a bench under a pullup bar and use it to boost your body so your chin is above the bar. Then take the prescribed amount of time—either 5 to 6 seconds or 8 to 10 seconds—to lower your body. Once your arms are straight, jump back up to the top position and repeat. Rest for 60 seconds after each set.

Week 1: Chinup: 3 sets: 5–6 reps: 5–6 seconds

Week 2: Neutral-grip pullup: 3 sets: 5–6 reps: 5–6 seconds

Week 3: Neutral-grip pullup: 2 sets: 5–6 reps: 8–10 seconds

Week 4: Pullup: 2 sets: 5–6 reps: 8–10 seconds

YOUR BEST EFFORT: 2 TO 4

The problem: You can't do enough repetitions to fully develop your mind-muscle connection, limiting your ability to become stronger.

The fix: Do more sets of fewer repetitions.

The reason: The first 1 or 2 repetitions in a set are the "highest quality" ones, meaning that's when the most muscle fibers fire. By doing several sets of 1 or 2 repetitions, you'll activate more total fibers and better develop the communication pathways between your brain and muscle—increasing strength quickly.

How to do it: Take the number of pullups you can complete and divide it by two. That's how many repetitions you'll do each set. (If your best effort is 3, round down to 1.) Follow the workout routine below, doing the number of sets indicated and resting for the prescribed amount of time after each. Note that after 2 weeks, you'll increase the repetitions you do in each set.

Week 1: 8 sets: 50 percent of best effort: 90 seconds rest

Week 2: 8 sets: 50 percent of best effort: 60 seconds rest

Week 3: 8 sets: Best effort: 90 seconds rest

Week 4: 8 sets: Best effort: 60 seconds rest

YOUR BEST EFFORT: 5 TO 7

The problem: You have strength but lack muscular endurance.

The fix: Focus on doing more total repetitions than normal—regardless of the number of sets it takes. For instance, instead of doing 3 sets of 6, for a total of 18 repetitions, you'll shoot for 30 repetitions—even if that means you have to drop down to sets of 3, 2, or 1. This will rapidly improve your muscular endurance.

How to do it: Perform as many pullups as you can, then rest for 60 seconds. Repeat as many times as needed to do 30 repetitions. Each workout, try to reach your goal in fewer sets.

YOUR BEST EFFORT: 8 TO 12

The problem: You're too strong for your body weight.

The fix: Make yourself heavier by doing pullups with added weight. You'll boost your absolute strength, which increases the number you can do with just your body weight.

How to do it: Attach a weight plate to a dipping belt and strap it around your waist. (If your gym doesn't have one, you can hold a dumbbell between your ankles.) Use a weight that's about 5 to 10 percent of your body weight, just enough so you'll be doing only 2 or 3 fewer repetitions than your best effort. Do 4 or 5 sets, resting 60 seconds after each.

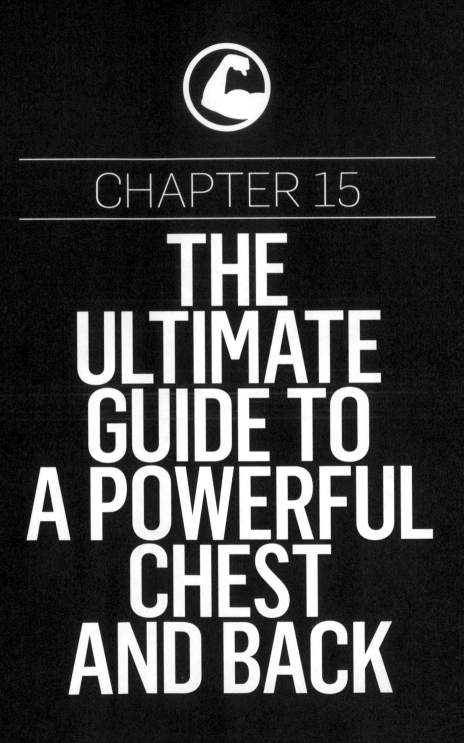

CHAPTER 15

THE ULTIMATE GUIDE TO A POWERFUL CHEST AND BACK

PART ONE

BUILD A BULLETPROOF CHEST

Guys tend to abandon the pushup for the bench press sometime around puberty. Which is why you usually have to wait in line at the gym for a bench while there's always plenty of floor space. But the once-forgotten pushup has recently muscled its way back to the top of the exercise universe. Why? Because it not only builds a powerful front façade to your physique but also develops the support system behind that musculature. "They're also a great way to judge how strong you are relative to your body weight," says Martin Rooney, P.T., C.S.C.S., author of *Ultimate Warrior Workouts*.

Test yourself by doing as many pushups as you can in 3 minutes. Rest whenever you want, but keep the clock running the whole time. Fifty-five is average, but if you can't reach 75—what strength coaches consider "good"—then you need to either gain strength or lose weight. Our 14 pushup variations will help you do both. Weave them into your daily workouts to build strength, power, and sleeve-busting muscle.

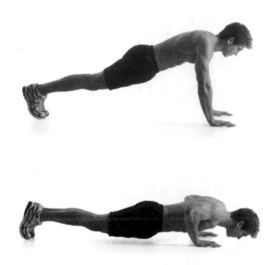

ROTATIONAL PUSHUP

Good for: Athletic performance in sports involving torso rotation, such as tennis, hockey, and baseball

Assume the classic pushup position, but as you come up, rotate your body so your right arm lifts up and extends overhead. Your arms and torso should form a T. Return to the starting position, lower yourself, then push up and rotate till your left hand points toward the ceiling.

Variations: One-dumbbell (grip a dumbbell in one hand, rotate to the dumbbell side for half your repetitions, then switch the dumbbell to the other hand); two-dumbbell (grip dumbbells in both hands, and alternate sides when you come up).

THE CLASSIC

Good for: General upper-body conditioning

Balance your weight on your toes and palms, with your hands a comfortable distance apart, probably just beyond shoulder-width. Your body should form a straight line from your ankles to your head. Squeeze your glutes and brace your abdominals, and keep them that way for the duration of the exercise. Slowly lower yourself to the floor, pause, and push yourself back up. Repeat a few hundred times.

Variations: Three-point pushup (place one foot on top of the other to make the exercise a little more challenging); decline pushup (set your feet on a bench or chair to strengthen your shoulders); and triceps pushup (place your hands close together, directly under your shoulders, and keep your elbows tucked close to your sides as you lower your body— an adjustment that shifts the work from your chest to your arms).

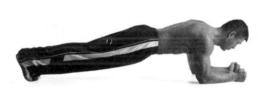

PLANK

Good for: Posture; midsection endurance, and stability

Lie facedown, rest your weight on your fore-arms and toes, tuck your hips, and hold your body in a straight line from ankles to shoulders for 5 seconds. Do a total of 10 5-second holds.

Variations: When 5-second holds are easy, progress to longer holds, until you can stay in the position for 30 seconds. Next, try a regular pushup position with your hips tucked. When you can hold that for 30 seconds, try it on your knuckles.

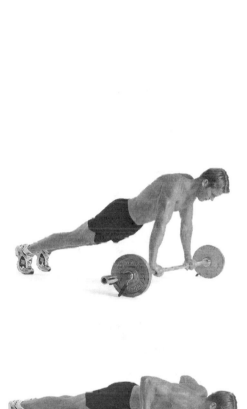

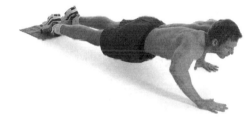

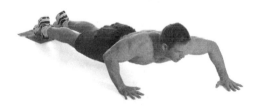

BARBELL PUSHUP
Good for: Stability of midsection, shoulder; grip strength
Get into the classic pushup position with your hands on a barbell (the kind that can roll away if you don't keep it steady). Knock out the pushups, but not yourself—keep in mind that one slip can send you crashing teeth-first into the floor.

WALKING PUSHUP
Good for: Abdominal development; shoulder stability
Set up in the classic pushup position on a smooth floor, and place your feet on a towel. Walk with your hands across the room, turn, and walk back. Keep your back flat throughout the movement.

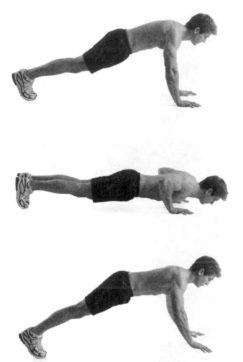

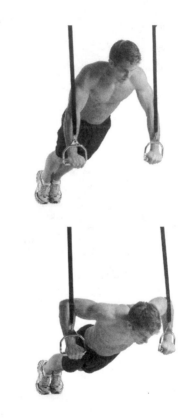

PLYOMETRIC PUSHUP
Good for: Developing upper-body power

Set up in the classic position on a well-padded carpet or exercise mat. Push up hard enough for your hands to come off the floor and catch some air. When you hit the floor, go immediately into the next repetition, pushing up again as hard as you can and catching more air.

SUSPENDED PUSHUP
Good for: Upper-body strength and stability

Wrap a pair of straps (or chains) around a chinup bar or the crossbar of a power rack. At the bottom, the straps should be about 12 inches off the floor. Attach gymnastics-type rings (or a straight bar) to the ends of the straps. Grab the rings and do pushups, being careful to protect your lower back by keeping your core and glutes tight—as you should when you do any variation of the pushup.

PART TWO

BUILD A BROADER BACK

The secret to a bigger, stronger back: Quit thinking of it as one big slab of muscle. Unlike your chest, your back is made up of more than just one major muscle group—it has lots of them. In fact, this hard-to-see part of your upper body houses a complex system of muscles, from your lats to your rotator cuffs to your upper, middle, and lower traps, with each area performing a variety of functions. That's why sculpting a V-shaped torso isn't as simple as doing "back" exercises, such as chinups and lat pulldowns. What's more, you probably need to play catch-up. After all, how many men spend as much time on their back muscles as they do on their pecs? To help you broaden your shoulders, thicken your lats, and beef up your traps, Bill Hartman, P.T., C.S.C.S., has identified five key back-building obstacles and their fixes. Apply them, and you'll experience gains in size and strength like never before.

YOUR UPPER BACK IS TIGHT.

When you spend a lot of time in one position—sitting at your desk, for example—the muscles of your upper back stiffen, which can lead to poor posture, weak shoulders, and neck and back pain.

YOU HAVEN'T MASTERED THE DEADLIFT.

If you allow your lower back to round when you deadlift—as most guys do—you place your lumbar spine in danger. Trouble is, many men are too weak to keep their lower back naturally arched—the key to safe lifting—as they lift the bar from the floor.

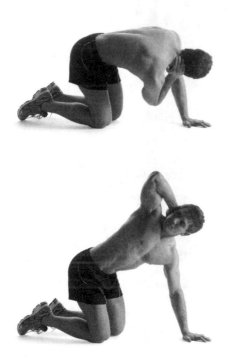

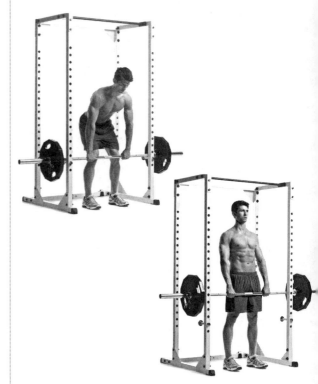

1. THORACIC ROTATION

Kneel down, place your right hand behind your head, and point your elbow out to the side. Brace your core and rotate your right shoulder toward your left arm. Follow your elbow with your eyes as you reverse the movement until your right elbow points toward the ceiling. That's 1 repetition. Do 20. After you've completed the prescribed number of reps, switch arms and repeat.

2. RACK PULL

Set a barbell at knee level in a squat rack. Assume a shortstop stance—your hips back, knees slightly bent, and knees against the bar. Your lower back should be naturally arched. Now grab the bar overhand with your hands just outside your legs. Stand up by pushing your hips forward. Begin with no weight until the exercise feels natural, and then start adding weight. Once the exercise becomes easy from the rack, lift the barbell from the floor using the same form.

YOUR ROWS MISS THE BOAT.

The row is a great exercise for your middle traps and rear shoulders, but only if you do it right. Many men lift with just their arm muscles instead of working their traps and rear delts.

YOU HAVE A GLARING WEAK SPOT.

Most men have weak scapular muscles, which stabilize your shoulder blades and provide the foundation for every upper-body lift. If these muscles are weak, your ability to lift more weight on exercises such as the bench press will suffer.

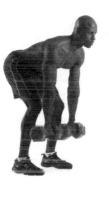

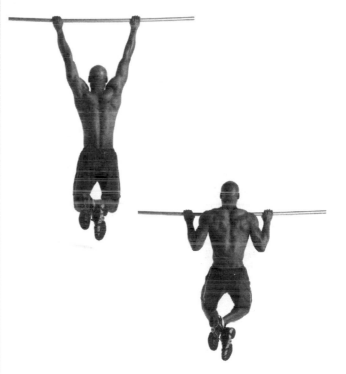

3B. TWO-PART DUMBBELL ROW

Grab a pair of dumbbells, bend at your hips and knees, and lower your torso until it's almost parallel to the floor. Let the weights hang at arm's length from your shoulders. First pull your shoulders back and hold that position. Then pull the weights to the sides of your torso by squeezing your shoulder blades toward your spine. Lower to the starting position and repeat.

See page 165 for Exercises 3A and 4A.

4B. PULLUP HOLD

Hang from a pullup bar with an overhand grip, your hands at the exact width you use when you do a bench press. Pull your chest up to the bar and hold for 10 to 20 seconds. Once you can do more than 5 reps, add resistance with a weighted vest or a dumbbell between your feet, or do regular pullups.

YOUR TRAPS ARE TOP-HEAVY.

Shrugs build your upper trapezius muscle, making it too strong relative to the middle and lower sections. This can cause shoulder impingement, a painful condition in which the muscles and tendons in your rotator cuff become pinched by your shoulder joint.

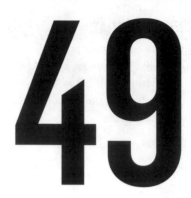

49

Percentage of men who perform crunches at least once a week

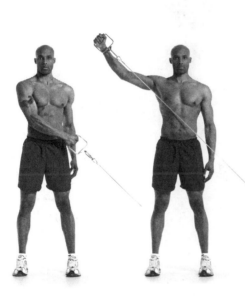

5. CABLE DIAGONAL RAISE

Attach a handle to the low pulley of a cable station. Standing with your left side toward the pulley, grab the handle with your right hand in front of your left hip and bend your elbow slightly. Pull the handle up and across your body until your hand is over your head and your thumb is pointing up (a Statue of Liberty pose). Return to the starting position. Complete all reps and repeat with your left arm.

The Ultimate Back Workout

Too much chest work overtrains the muscles on your front, leaving your back vulnerable to injury. Turn your workout around with this plan.

Complete this upper-body workout twice a week, resting at least 3 days between sessions. Do the exercises in the order shown, using the heaviest weight that allows you to complete the prescribed number of reps. Perform exercises 1, 2, and 5 as straight sets, completing all sets of each exercise before moving on. Do exercises 3A and 3B, and exercises 4A and 4B, as alternating sets. That is, do 1 set of 3A, rest for 1 to 2 minutes, do 1 set of 3B, and rest again. Repeat until you've done all sets of both exercises. Use the same procedure for 4A and 4B.

EXERCISE	SETS	REPS	REST (MIN.)
1. Thoracic rotation	2	20	1
2. Rack pull	3	6	2–4
3A. Dumbbell bench press (see below)	3	8–10	1–2
3B. Two-part dumbbell row	3	8–10	1–2
4A. Alternating dumbbell shoulder press (see below)	3	8–10	1–2
4B. Pullup hold	3	3–5	1–2
5. Cable diagonal raise	2	10–12	1

3A. DUMBBELL BENCH PRESS

Grab a pair of dumbbells and lie on your back on a flat bench, holding the dumbbells over your chest so they're nearly touching. Lower the dumbbells to the side of your chest. Pause, then press the weights back up to the starting positional as quickly as you can. That's 1 rep.

4A. ALTERNATING DUMBBELL SHOULDER PRESS

Stand holding a pair of dumbbells just outside your shoulders, with your arms bent and palms facing each other. Press your right hand upward until your arm is completely straight. Slowly lower the dumbbell back to the starting position. Continue with your left hand, alternating with each rep.

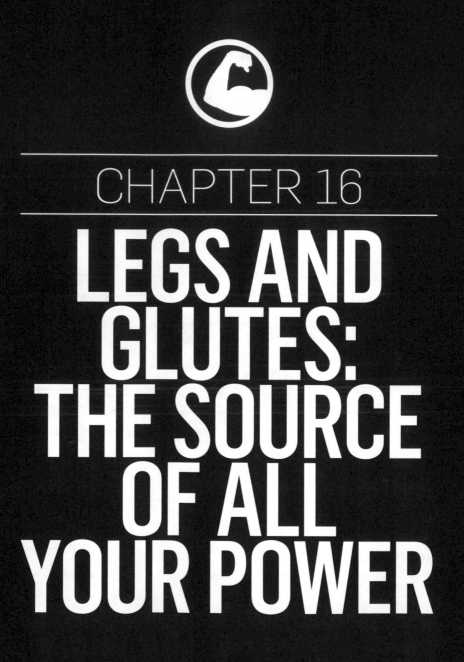

CHAPTER 16

LEGS AND GLUTES: THE SOURCE OF ALL YOUR POWER

When it comes to lifting weights, it's tempting to skip your lower body. After all, we wear pants to work. But that half-assed approach (or all-ass, since you're ignoring your glutes as well) limits the amount of muscle you can add to your body by at least 50 percent. Do the math.

The good news: You're only one step away from dramatic improvements. That's because you can adopt the unique leg workout that Martin Rooney, P.T., C.S.C.S., gives to athletes training for the NFL combine. By shocking your wheels with this plan, you'll pack on pounds of muscle, burn tons of calories, and raise your game in every sport. And that'll give you a leg up on looking better all over.

THE WORKOUT

Use this two-part routine 3 days a week, resting at least a day between sessions. Do workout A, which is designed to enhance speed and explosiveness, twice a week. Do workout B once a week to build size and strength. Always sandwich workout B between your workout As. A good strategy: Do workout A when you train your upper body, and workout B on a day all by itself. (Yes, it's that challenging.)

WORKOUT A: POWER

Perform 3 sets of 6 reps of each exercise, resting 60 seconds between sets. Move as quickly as possible while maintaining proper form.

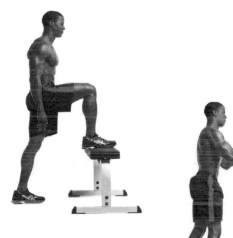

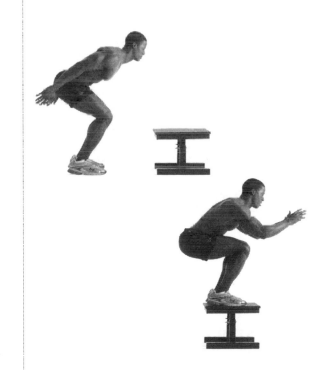

EXPLOSIVE STEPUP

Perform a stepup with dumbbells, but explosively swing your arms into the air and jump up, landing back on the box or bench on one foot. Slowly lower your body back to the floor. That's 1 rep. Do all your reps on one leg, and then repeat with the opposite leg.

BENCH JUMP

Stand facing the bench in quarter-squat position. Bend your knees slightly, and then jump up. Land as softly as possible by bending your knees. Step down and repeat.

WORKOUT A (continued)

WORKOUT B: SIZE AND STRENGTH

Perform 3 sets of 6 to 8 repetitions of each exercise, resting 2 to 3 minutes between sets. On every exercise, focus on taking 2 to 3 seconds to lower your body. To make the movements more difficult, add resistance by holding a dumbbell in each hand.

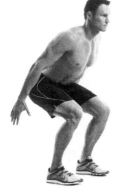

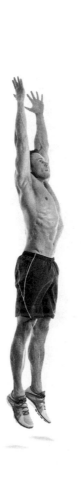

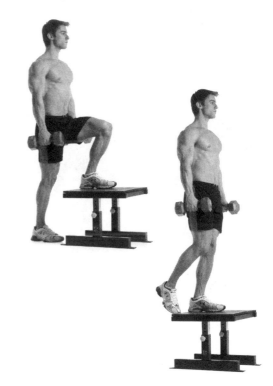

SQUAT JUMP

Stand as tall as you can. Dip your knees and squat down, swinging your arms back in preparation to leap. Explosively jump as high as you can. When you land immediately squat down and jump again.

STEPUP

Grab a pair of dumbbells. Stand 6 to 8 inches from a box, and place your right foot on top of it. Press through your right heel and step onto the box or bench, but don't let your left foot touch the box. Slowly lower your left foot back to the floor. That's 1 rep. Do all reps on your right leg, and then switch legs and repeat.

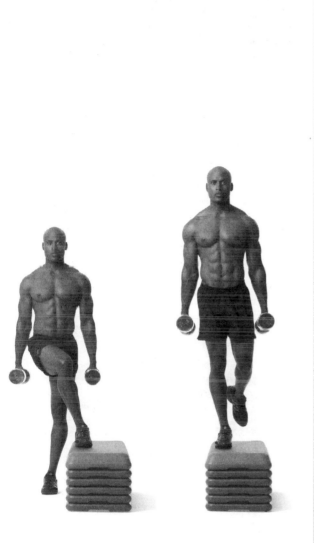

CROSSOVER STEPUP

Grab a pair of dumbbells and stand with a box to your left. Place your right foot on top of it, with your right knee bent 90 degrees. Push yourself up with your right leg, keeping your left foot off the box. Pause, and reverse the motion. Do all reps on your right leg, and then turn around to switch to your left.

STEPUP WITH STRAIGHT-LEG DEADLIFT

Perform a stepup with your right leg. Once you're on top of the box or bench, bend your hips while maintaining a slight bend in your right knee, and lower your torso until it's almost parallel to the floor. Pause, and slowly raise your torso back up and step back down to the floor. That's 1 rep. Complete all reps on your right leg, and then switch legs and repeat.

WORKOUT B (continued)

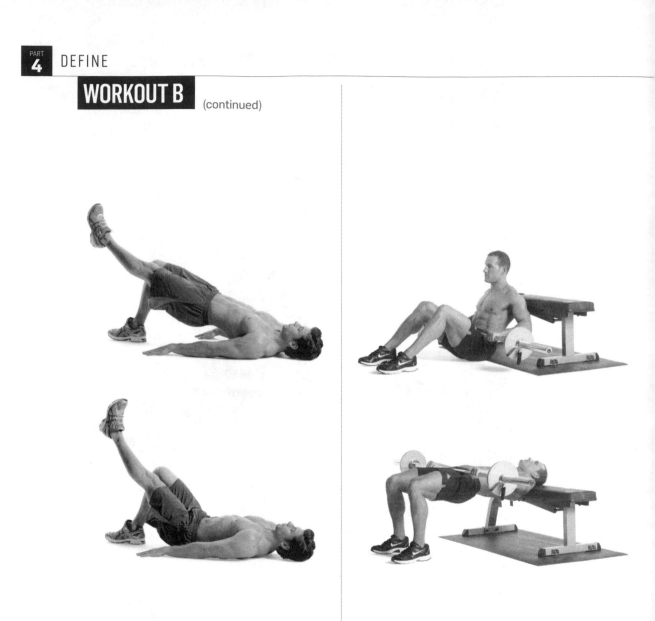

SINGLE-LEG HIP RAISE

Lie on your back with your left heel raised and your left knee straight. Your right knee should be bent 90 degrees and your right foot flat on the floor. Lift your hips so your body forms a straight line from your shoulders to your right knee. Slowly lower your body. Complete all your reps, switch legs, and repeat.

BARBELL HIP THRUST

Place your upper back against a box or bench with your knees bent and feet flat on the floor. Put a padded barbell across your hips so your glutes are near the floor. Then squeeze your glutes and raise your hips until they're in line with your body. Return to the starting position, and repeat.

Check the height of your box: Your knee should form about a 90-degree angle when you place that foot on top of the box.

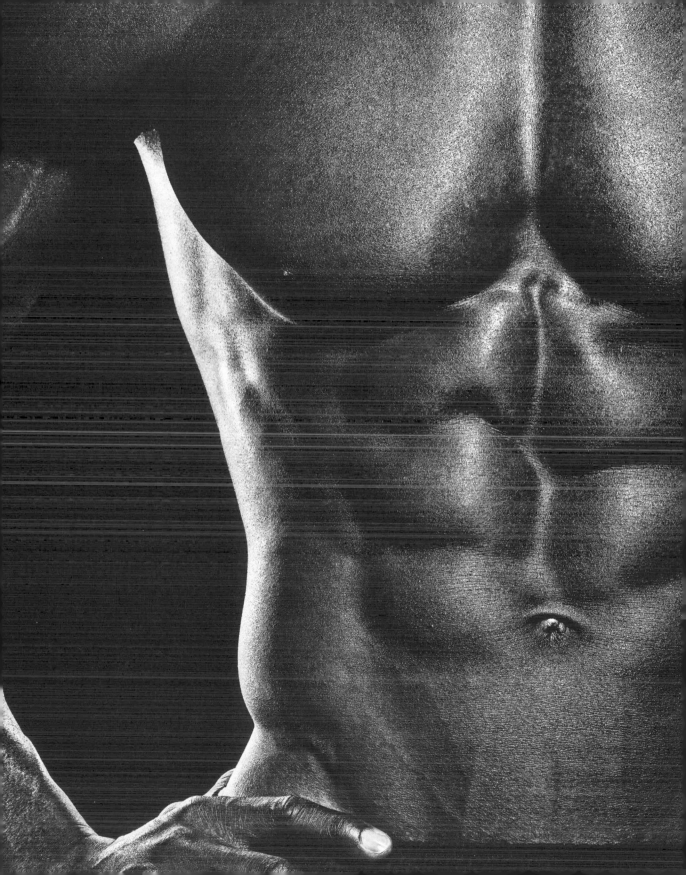

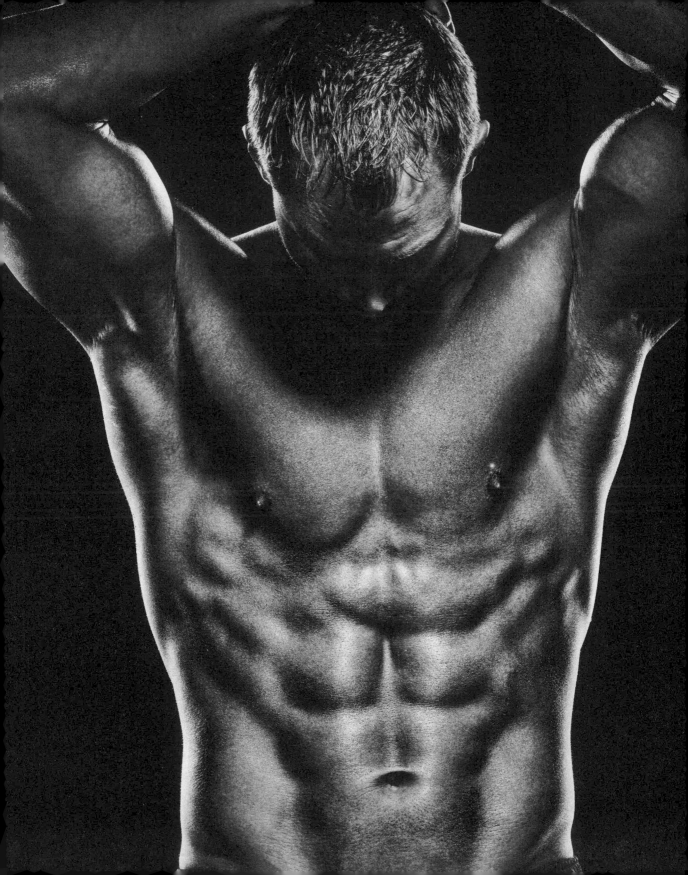

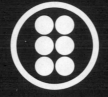

PART FIVE

CUT

THE SIMPLE SECRETS TO SIX-PACK ABS

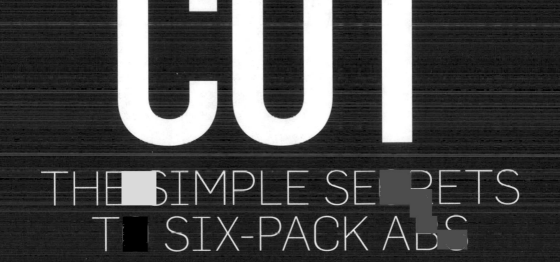

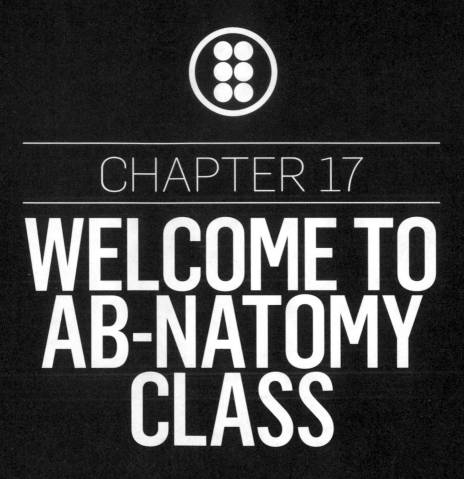

CHAPTER 17

WELCOME TO AB-NATOMY CLASS

THE FIRST STEP TO A SIX-PACK IS UNDERSTANDING YOUR ABS.

Knowledge is power, after all. So consider this chapter Ab-natomy 101.

THE ANATOMY OF YOUR SIX-PACK (TO BE UNCOVERED)

Your abdominal muscles are a lot like employees—not the ones goofing off on Facebook or taking 2-hour business lunches. We're talking about the dedicated ones who give their all. Like employees, the harder your abs work, the better they make you look, and vice versa. This is because you use your abs in virtually every movement that matters. Lifting. Running. Jumping. Reproducing. (It takes a lot of midsection stability to stand over that copy machine. Especially when it's printing on both sides of the page.) So the stronger they are, the harder and longer you'll be able to play and the better you'll look while playing. Here's a quick course in the anatomy of your abs. You need to understand what you're after. If you can visualize them, you can find them. Your abs are made up of three main muscle groups:

Rectus abdominis. This is the six-pack muscle that helps your upper body bend (like in a crunch) and also helps maintain good posture. A long sheet of muscle running from your sternum to your pubic bone, it's what people think of when they think of abs. The ideal rectus abdominis has six segments of muscle above the belly button. This is the upper abs, or what most of us refer to as the six-pack. Then there's a flat sheath below the belly button that forms the lower abs. Still, it's one long sheet of muscle. There are a lot of different looks when it comes to six-packs. Some folks have segments aligned symmetrically; others are asymmetric. Some people have a four-pack or a six-pack, and some lucky ones even have an eight-pack. It all depends on your genetic makeup. But no matter what you have undercover now, you should take a bow when you are able to see exactly what kind you have when you take off your shirt. Abs take work to unveil.

Obliques. You have two types, external and internal. Your obliques frame your rectus abdominis, create shape in your torso from hips to chest, and act as a postural muscle to keep your torso straight. Each type has an assigned duty:

External. These are the muscles that help you twist at the waist. They start on the ribs and extend diagonally down the sides of your waist. If a movement happens at your waist, the external obliques are involved. The torso rotation that's key to golf, tennis, and hockey is mostly a function of the external obliques. Even the basic crunching motion, attributed to the rectus abdominis (the six-pack muscle), wouldn't be possible without a strong contraction of the external obliques to stabilize the torso.

Internal. These lie between the rib cage and the external obliques, and also extend diagonally down the sides of your waist. Similar to the externals, the internal obliques are involved in torso rotation and posture. You use these muscles when you breathe deeply.

Transverse abdominis. It's a thin muscle that runs horizontally, underneath your rectus abdominis and obliques and surrounding your abdomen. Your deepest abdominal muscle, it's also known as "the girdle" because it pulls your abdominal wall inward—as when you're sucking in your gut—and keeps everything in place.

MORE ON YOUR CORE

Technically, the rectus abdominis, obliques, and transverse abdominis make up your abs. But there's more to your core. Actually, the term *core* describes the entire complex of spine stabilizers, more than two dozen abdominal, lower-back, and hip muscles that keep your torso upright and allow you to rotate, bend forward, backward, and from side to side. Let's take a look at the non-abs muscles that contribute to your core.

Hip flexors. This group of muscles is found on the front of your hips. Originating on either your spine or pelvis, they make up the ground floor of your core. Your main hip flexors are the tensor fasciae latae, psoas, and iliacus. Their job is to allow your hips to flex, as their name suggests. When you run or raise your upper legs to your chest, you are calling on your hip flexors to do the job.

Lower back. There are many lower-back muscles that contribute to your core strength, but the main ones are your spinal erectors, technically called your erector spinae, multifidus, and quadratus lumborum. These muscles of the lower back are attached to another muscle complex called the gluteus maximus. We mention it here because your glutes or butt muscles work in conjunction with these core muscles. Collectively, these muscles help keep your spine stable and also allow it to bend backward and to the side.

Nobody starts an exercise program with hopes of getting great-looking spinal erectors or hip flexors, but these muscles are crucial to your day-to-day feelings of health and vitality. Sitting all day weakens the muscles and stretches out the connective tissues in your lower back, making you feel drained when you get home. Strengthening your lower back and abdominals in tandem will improve your posture, make sitting more comfortable, and leave you with energy at the end of the day.

Three Things You Don't Know about Your Abs

1. **You can strengthen your core without moving a muscle.** Whereas most muscles propel you, your core resists movement—for instance, to protect your spine when you twist your torso. So don't be surprised by how hard it is to do the stability exercises in this section.

2. **Slouching sabotages your six-pack.** Training your core helps correct poor posture. But an hour a week of core can't compensate for the 50 hours you spend slumped over your keyboard. The fix: Stay tall through your hips, and keep your head up and shoulder blades back and down all day long.

3. **Core muscles contract first in every exercise.** All the energy you exert originates in your torso before being transferred to your arms and legs. So a weak core reduces the amount of force you're able to apply to a barbell. When you hit a plateau in presses, squats, or any other strength move, ask yourself if you're training your core as hard as you can.

SIX HABITS FOR A SIX-PACK

If you can't see your abs, don't assume it's because you're missing out on a magical abdominal exercise or secret supplement. Blame your mindset.

You see, losing belly flab is a boring process. It requires time, hard work, and, most important, dedication. Take the right steps every single day, and you'll ultimately carve out your six-pack. But if you stray from your plan even a few times a week—which most men do—you'll probably never see your abs.

The solution: six simple habits that can help you strip away your lard for good. Think of these habits as daily goals designed to keep you on the fast track to a fit-looking physique. Individually they're not all that surprising, but together they become a powerful tool.

The effectiveness of this tool is even supported by science. At the University of Iowa, researchers determined that people are more likely to stick with their fat-loss plans when they concentrate on specific actions instead of the desired result. So rather than focusing on abs that show, follow this daily list of nutrition, exercise, and lifestyle strategies for achieving that rippled midsection. The result: automatic abs.

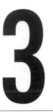

WAKE UP TO WATER.

Imagine not drinking all day at work—no coffee, no water, no diet soda. At the end of an 8-hour shift, you'd be pretty parched. Which is precisely why you should start rehydrating immediately after a full night's slumber. From now on, drink at least 16 ounces of chilled H_2O as soon as you rise in the morning. German scientists recently found that doing this boosts metabolism by 24 percent for 90 minutes afterward. (A smaller amount of water had no effect.) What's more, a previous study determined that muscle cells grow faster when they're well hydrated. A general rule of thumb: Guzzle at least a gallon of water over the course of a day.

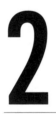

EAT BREAKFAST EVERY DAY.

Do this for the same reason in number 1. Your body hasn't had food in 8 hours, so fuel up and help yourself stay lean. A University of Massachusetts study showed that men who skip their morning meal are $4\frac{1}{2}$ times more likely to be overweight than those who don't. So within an hour of waking, have a meal or protein shake with at least 250 calories, and cap your intake at 500 calories. For a quick way to fuel up first thing, try this recipe: Prepare a package of instant oatmeal and mix in a scoop of whey protein powder and $\frac{1}{2}$ cup of blueberries.

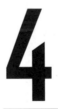

AS YOU EAT, REVIEW YOUR GOALS...

It's important that you stay aware of your mission. University of Iowa scientists found that people who monitored their diet and exercise goals most frequently were more likely to achieve them than were goal setters who rarely reviewed their objectives.

... AND THEN PACK YOUR LUNCH.

This habit should be as much a part of your morning ritual as showering. Use a small personal cooler to keep the foods you need within arm's reach, thus preventing all the other lousy food around you from finding its way into your hands, and then your mouth. Some unbelievably simple suggestions:

- An apple (to eat as a morning snack)
- Two slices of cheese (to eat with the apple)
- A 500- to 600-calorie portion of leftovers (for your lunch)
- A premixed protein shake or a pint of milk (for your afternoon snack)

By using this approach, you'll keep your body well fed and satisfied throughout the day without overeating. You'll also provide your body with the nutrients it needs for your workout, no matter what time you exercise. Just as important, you'll be much less likely to be tempted by the office candy bowl. And you can make this rule even simpler: Don't eat anything that's not in the cooler.

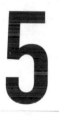

EXERCISE THE RIGHT WAY.

Everyone has abs, even if people can't always see them because they're hidden under a layer of flab. That means you don't need to do endless crunches to carve out a six-pack. Instead, you should spend most of your gym time burning off blubber.

The most effective strategy is a one-two approach of weight lifting and high-intensity interval training. According to a recent University of Southern Maine study, half an hour of pumping iron burns as many calories as running at a 6-minute-per-mile pace for the same duration. (And it has the added benefit of helping you build muscle.)

What's more, unlike aerobic exercise, lifting has been shown to boost metabolism for as long as 39 hours after the last repetition. Similar findings have been noted for intervals, which are short, all-out sprints interspersed with periods of rest.

For the best results, do a total-body weight-training workout 3 days a week, resting at least a day between sessions. Then do an interval-training session on the days in between. (See Chapter 19 for a terrific fat-burning plan.)

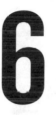

SKIP THE LATE SHOWS.

You need sleep to unveil your six-pack. That's because lack of shut-eye may disrupt the hormones that control your ability to burn fat. For instance, University of Chicago scientists recently found that just 3 nights of poor sleep may cause your muscle cells to become resistant to the hormone insulin. Over time, this leads to fat storage around your belly.

To achieve a better night's sleep, review your goals again 15 minutes before bedtime. And while you're at it, write down your plans for the next day's work schedule, as well as any personal chores you need to accomplish. This can help prevent you from lying awake worrying about tomorrow ("I have to remember to e-mail Johnson"), which can cut into quality snooze time.

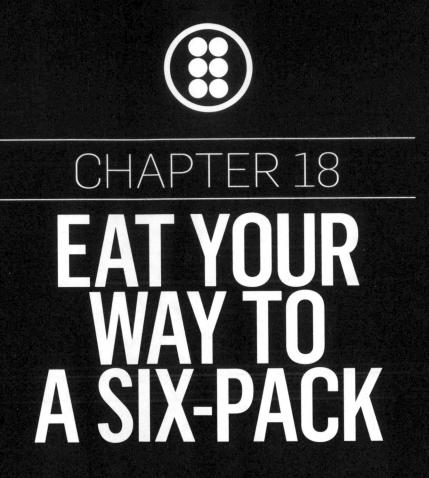

CHAPTER 18

EAT YOUR WAY TO A SIX-PACK

The fix to all of your dieting woes can be solved in one sentence: *Stop looking for a one-size-fits-all solution.* That was the message of a 20-year study on weight loss conducted at the Harvard School of Public Health. The researchers concluded that dieters who focused only on how much they ate—rather than the types of foods they consumed—were more likely to fail at losing weight.

The reason: Restrictive dieting isn't sustainable and causes stress, which increases the likelihood of long-term failure. That's not to say that removing certain foods doesn't work. Or that counting calories isn't an effective way to easily drop pounds. It is. In fact, it's so effective that a Kansas State University professor proved that by counting calories, he could eat a diet consisting of Twinkies and chips and still lose 27 pounds—in just 2 months! (Take that, Slim-Fast!) The experiment showed that how much food you consume is still the most important factor in the weight-loss equation. It also proved that any food—if you can call Twinkies food (they have more than 40 ingredients and can survive multiple apocalypses)—could be part of a weight-loss plan. And while the empty-calorie diet might leave your taste buds satisfied and your buddies impressed, it won't help you live longer, fight aging, and build muscle. Your goal isn't to minimize how much food you eat. It's to make sure you're filling your body with quality foods that will help you lose weight *and* add healthy, nutritional benefits.

If you want to experience success like never before, all you have to do is make three simple promises to yourself. Say 'em out loud. Learn 'em by heart. Then use them as you eat your way through the 4-week six-pack nutrition plan that follows.

"I WILL EAT GREENS. EVERY. DAY."
Here's a rule you probably never thought you'd hear suggested in a diet plan: Eat as much as you want. But that's exactly what you can do with vegetables. Whether you prefer spinach, peppers, asparagus, or exotic offerings like bok choy and kale,

pack your plate high with as many shades of green and varieties as you like. Vegetables are packed with so many supernutrients that they have been linked to almost every health benefit imaginable—heart health, cancer prevention, a boost in mood and energy, even revving up your sex life.

The biggest benefit, however, is weight loss. A study in the *American Journal of Clinical Nutrition* found that men who included veggies in every meal were able to eat 25 percent more food but lose an additional 3.5 pounds. How? Vegetables help you lose fat by keeping you more satisfied, so you're less likely to overeat. (And they have fewer calories.) Greens are low in calories, high in volume, and nutrient dense. So you can eat a lot of them, feel full, and not have to worry about other foods sneaking into your diet and sinking your healthy eating plan.

"I WILL MAKE PROTEIN MY WINGMAN."
When it comes to ripped abs, protein is your secret weapon When you consider that Johns Hopkins University linked a high-protein diet to lower blood pressure, less body fat, better cholesterol levels, improved triglycerides, and the prevention of diabetes, obesity, and osteoporosis, it's no wonder we're in favor of protein. But if you're like most men—even those who love steak and wings—you're not doing a good enough job using this crucial weight-loss tool.
Your plan of attack: Eat protein in every meal and snack. Focusing on protein fights off hunger and makes your stomach unlikely to bulge since protein is less likely to be stored as fat. That's because protein is harder to digest, so you burn more calories

just eating the food. This process also helps ensure you eat less. Men who made sure their diet was at least 30 percent protein ate almost 450 calories less per day and lost 11 pounds *more* than those who ate less protein, according to a study published in *Nutrition & Metabolism.*

So whether it's burgers, chicken, or eggs, you'll be eating a constant source of nature's ultimate abs superfood.

"I WILL TRADE EMPTY CALORIES FOR *REAL* CARBS."

If there's one "food group" you should limit on this plan, it's sugar. Your fix: Eat more fruit. Fruit—nature's sweet reward—provides plenty of carbs for energy, but has less impact on your blood sugar than processed sweets and other carbohydrates. This is crucial to help you avoid the cravings and binges that occur when your blood sugar rises quickly and then crashes. Ideally, the majority of your carbs will come from fruits. That doesn't mean you won't have grains, beans, or other carbohydrate sources and the occasional treat. Limit yourself to just a couple servings daily of sugars and processed carbohydrate sources, and consume the rest of your carbs from fresh produce. You'll soon find you don't even miss your old sugary snacks.

SO ... WHAT SHOULD YOU EAT?

In the following plan, you'll eat three main meals per day (breakfast, lunch, dinner) plus additional snacks. You can eat the snacks as separate meals, or you can add them to any of the main eating times to create a bigger meal. Finally—an eating plan where *you* are in control.

Five Ways to Eat Less

1. **Use smaller utensils.** According to a University of Rhode Island at Kingston study, people who opted for the smaller cutlery consumed 70 calories less per meal.

2. **Eat slower.** When you take more time to chew (think breaking your meal down into particles), you're able to savor the texture and taste of food. Not only will this make your meal more enjoyable, it gives your body the time it needs to register a full belly (generally 15 to 20 minutes). Those who eat quickly tend to pack in more food.

3. **Be a social eater.** This goes with number 2 above. If you talk to your friends or family when you eat, you prolong the length of your meal. The longer your meal lasts, the less likely you are to overeat. Plus, the mental distraction helps prevent overindulging, according to researchers at Flinders University.

4. **Make it a hot meal.** Apparently, your stomach likes it hot—as in hot sauce. Adding spices to your meal helps you chew your food more thoroughly and drink more water—one of the keys to a better eating plan.

5. **End with black tea.** The green version might receive all the love, but black tea actually decreases your blood sugar after a meal for up to 2.5 hours, according to a study in the *Journal of the American College of Nutrition*. The benefit: You'll feel fuller faster and stay satisfied longer.

BREAKFAST

Breakfast is designed to get you started off on the right food. That means a plentiful offering of dairy options like yogurt or milk, protein from eggs or a protein smoothie, and your choice of grains or fruit.

LUNCH

The foundation of lunch is lean protein like chicken or tuna. Combine that with your favorite vegetables or a side salad to help you power through your afternoon.

DINNER

Your evening meal is packed with more protein, but this time you can go for something a little fattier, like steak, salmon, or trout. These fats will help you stay full. Once again, pile your plate high with veggies, such as grilled zucchini, asparagus, and squash, or sauté some spinach and broccoli.

SNACKS

This is where the fun begins and you really take control of your daily menu. Remember, snacks can be eaten separately at any point in the day, or they can be added to any meal. Each day, add healthy fat sources like nuts, a small source of protein such as deli meat, and some smart carbs like a piece of fruit or grains such as a bowl of cereal.

Substitutions? Of Course!

YOUR FLEXIBLE EATING GUIDE

The 4-week eating plan will put you on the fast track to six-pack abs. But that doesn't mean you can't make substitutions and eat *your* way, every day. Here's a quick cheat sheet that you can use to fuel your body with any food choice. Use "The Lean Guide Shopping List" (next page) and apply your favorite foods.

MEAL 1	MEAL 2	MEAL 3	SNACKS (eat separately or add to any meal)
2–3 servings protein	2–3 servings protein	3 servings protein	2–3 servings protein
1 serving dairy	Unlimited vegetables	1–2 servings healthy fat/nuts	1 serving healthy fat/nuts or 1 serving dairy
1 serving fruit or grain		Unlimited vegetables	2–3 servings fruit or starches/grains
Unlimited vegetables			

THE LEAN GUIDE

SHOPPING LIST

PROTEIN SOURCES
(serving size = 4 ounces)

Canned tuna

Chicken breast

Eggs

Fish (all types)

Lean ground beef

Lean pork (ham, bacon)

Lean turkey

Shrimp

DAIRY
(with serving size)

Cheese: 1 stick or slice

Cottage cheese (2% fat):
6 ounces

Milk (2% fat): 1 cup

Plain low-fat yogurt:
6 ounces (one single
serving of prepackaged)

STARCHES AND GRAINS
(with serving size)

Black beans: 1/2 cup

Bread (with 3 grams of
fiber or more): 1 slice

Cannellini beans: $1/2$ cup

Cereal (with 3 grams of
fiber or more): 1 cup

Corn tortillas: 1 tortilla

Flour tortillas (with 3 grams
of fiber or more): 1 tortilla

Garbanzo beans: $1/2$ cup

Oatmeal: $1/2$ cup

Pasta: $1/2$ cup (cooked)

Pita bread: 1 pita

Potatoes (regular or sweet):
1 medium-sized potato
(size of your fist)

FRUITS
Apples

Bananas

Blueberries

Cantaloupe

Grapefruit

Grapes

Kiwi

Orange

Peaches

Pears

Pineapple

Raspberries

Strawberries

Watermelon

FATS AND NUTS
Avocado:
$1/2$ tablespoon

Nut butters:
2 ounces

Almond

Cashew

Peanut

Nuts: a handful
(1 ounce)

Almonds

Brazil nuts

Cashews

Pecans

Pistachios

Walnuts

Sour cream:
2 tablespoons

VEGETABLES
(unlimited)

Artichokes

Arugula

Asparagus

Bell peppers

Bok choy

Broccoli

Cabbage

Carrots

Cauliflower

Celery

Cucumber

Green beans

Kale

Leafy greens

Leeks

Lettuce

Mushrooms

Onion

Spinach

Sprouts

Squash

Zucchini

YOUR 4-WEEK SIX-PACK EATING PLAN

WEEK 1

MONDAY

MEAL 1
- 1 cup plain Greek yogurt
- ½ cup blueberries
- ¼ cup sliced strawberries

MEAL 2
- 6 ounces sesame-crusted ahi tuna served over a bed of mixed greens, drizzled with balsamic vinaigrette

MEAL 3
- 6–8 ounces Cajun-rubbed top sirloin with grilled zucchini, onion, and steamed spinach

SNACKS
- Banana and almond butter
- 2–3 hard-cooked eggs

TUESDAY

MEAL 1
- Strawberry-Banana Protein Smoothie (Blend 1 banana, ½ cup strawberries, 1 cup almond milk, 1½ scoops vanilla whey protein powder, and 4 ice cubes.)

MEAL 2
- 6 ounces baked salmon with peach-mango salsa
- 1 cup sliced cantaloupe
- Steamed spinach

MEAL 3
- 6–8 ounces grilled chicken breast, cooked in olive oil, topped with ½ avocado
- Side of grilled asparagus and squash

SNACKS
- 1 apple
- 3 ounces hard cheese

WEDNESDAY

MEAL 1
- Mexican scrambled eggs (3 eggs, chopped tomatoes, onions, spinach, bell peppers, ½ cup shredded cheese, ¼ cup salsa)
- 1 orange

MEAL 2
- ½ cup shirataki noodles with 6 ounces ground turkey, roasted spinach, and mushrooms

MEAL 3
- Kebabs with 2 ounces shrimp, 6 ounces chicken, onion, and red and green bell peppers
- Kale salad topped with ½ avocado

SNACKS
- 1 cup cottage cheese
- 1 handful of almonds

THURSDAY

MEAL 1
- 2 slices whole grain toast
- 2 tablespoons almond butter
- 1 cup 1% milk

MEAL 2
- 6 ounces grilled chicken with arugula, baby spinach, walnuts, cucumbers, mint leaves, and mandarin oranges

MEAL 3
- 8 ounces grass-fed burger (less than 10% fat) with sautéed bell peppers, onions, and mushrooms

SNACKS
- 3 strips turkey jerky
- 1 stick mozzarella cheese

FRIDAY

MEAL 1
- Egg and cheese sandwich (Scramble 2 eggs, melt 1 slice of cheese, and place onto toasted English muffin.)

MEAL 2
- 6 ounces tuna steak marinated in 2 tablespoons soy sauce, 2 teaspoons wasabi, and 1 tablespoon rice wine vinegar
- Side salad with mixed greens, broccoli, and bell peppers

MEAL 3
- Turkey chili (8 ounces lean ground turkey, diced tomatoes, black beans, corn, dried chili mix, ground flaxseed, ¼ cup water)

SNACKS
- 1 can of tuna topped with salsa
- 1 handful of walnuts
- 1 apple

SATURDAY

MEAL 1
- Strawberry protein pancakes (Mix 1 scoop vanilla protein powder with 1 egg, ½ cup milk, ½ cup oats, 1 teaspoon salt, 1 teaspoon baking powder. Blend and pour on a griddle. Slice up 1 cup of strawberries and place atop the pancakes when done.)

MEAL 2
- Tuna melt sandwich (1 can tuna, 2 slices multigrain bread, ½ sliced avocado, 1 slice Cheddar cheese)

MEAL 3
- 6 ounces grilled chicken and steak skewers, mixed with bell peppers, onions, and zucchini

SNACKS
- Chocolate–Peanut Butter Smoothie (Blend 1 scoop chocolate protein powder, 1 tablespoon cocoa powder, 1 tablespoon peanut butter, 6 ounces almond milk, and 4 ice cubes.)

SUNDAY

MEAL 1
- Smoked salmon scramble (3 eggs, ¼ sliced onion, 3 ounces smoked salmon, capers)
- Grapefruit

MEAL 2
- 6 ounces seared trout topped with herbs and drizzled with olive oil
- Side of steamed broccoli

MEAL 3
- 8 ounces broiled salmon topped with lime, slow-roasted Roma tomatoes, and broccolini
- Spinach and kale salad

SNACKS
- 1 cup ice cream
- 1 cup mixed berries

YOUR 4-WEEK
SIX-PACK
EATING PLAN

WEEK

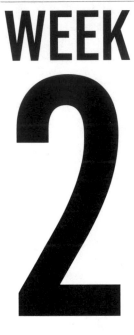

MONDAY

MEAL 1
3-egg omelet with spinach, mushrooms, onions, bell peppers, and Cheddar cheese

$\frac{1}{2}$ cup oatmeal topped with cinnamon

MEAL 2
6 ounces grilled chicken breasts marinated in 2 tablespoons teriyaki sauce and 1 tablespoon water

Side of roasted butternut squash and walnuts

MEAL 3
8 ounces pork chops glazed with Dijon mustard

Side of sweet potatoes and broccoli

SNACKS
1 cup plain Greek yogurt with $\frac{1}{2}$ cup blueberries and blackberries

1 handful of almonds

TUESDAY

MEAL 1
2 strips bacon and 2 fried eggs

Grapefruit

MEAL 2
Chicken fajitas (6 ounces sliced chicken breast, onion, green and red bell peppers, 1 jalapeño chile pepper, cilantro, cumin, 1 whole wheat tortilla)

MEAL 3
8 ounces cedar plank salmon seasoned with salt and pepper, and drizzled with olive oil

Side salad with cucumber, artichoke, broccoli, sprouts, and tomatoes

SNACKS
Chocolate–Peanut Butter Smoothie (Blend 1 scoop chocolate protein powder, 1 tablespoon cocoa powder, 1 tablespoon peanut butter, 6 ounces almond milk, and 4 ice cubes.)

WEDNESDAY

MEAL 1
Supercereal (cereal of choice with more than 3 grams of fiber, topped with sliced bananas and 1 tablespoon chia seeds)

3 hard-cooked eggs

MEAL 2
6 ounces grilled salmon with a spinach and arugula salad

MEAL 3
Turkey meatballs (8 ounces extra-lean ground turkey, 1 clove garlic, 4 saltine crackers, $\frac{1}{4}$ onion, $\frac{1}{4}$ cup tomato sauce)

Grilled bell peppers, butternut squash

SNACKS
1 cup plain cottage cheese

$\frac{1}{2}$ cantaloupe

1 handful of almonds

THURSDAY

MEAL 1

$\frac{1}{2}$ cup oatmeal, cinnamon, $\frac{1}{4}$ cup raisins

2–3 links chicken sausage

MEAL 2

Soba noodle chicken pad thai ($\frac{1}{4}$ cup soba noodles, 6 ounces chicken, peas, carrots, water chestnuts, and $\frac{1}{4}$ cup diced peanuts. Add a sauce of 2 teaspoons sriracha and 2 tablespoons soy sauce when finished cooking.)

MEAL 3

4 ounces grilled calamari and 4 ounces grilled shrimp served over sautéed Swiss chard and shallots

SNACKS

4 strips beef jerky

$\frac{1}{4}$ cup quinoa

FRIDAY

MEAL 1

Breakfast burrito (3 eggs scrambled, 1 whole grain tortilla, shredded mozzarella cheese, 2 ounces shredded chicken, sliced tomato, onions, bell peppers, avocado)

MEAL 2

6 ounces roasted halibut with $\frac{1}{2}$ cup fava beans, yellow squash, and shallot sauce

MEAL 3

Spicy beef and chicken stir-fry (4 ounces lean steak, 4 ounces chicken, spinach, bell peppers, onions, mushrooms, snap peas, bean sprouts, 2 tablespoons soy sauce, and as much sriracha as desired)

SNACKS

1 apple and 1 tablespoon almond butter

1 cup milk

SATURDAY

MEAL 1

Protein Berry Smoothie (Blend 2 scoops vanilla protein powder, 6 ounces almond milk, $\frac{1}{2}$ cup strawberries, $\frac{1}{2}$ cup blueberries, $\frac{1}{4}$ cup blackberries, 1 tablespoon chia seeds, 1 cup spinach, and 4 ice cubes.)

MEAL 2

Spinach wrap filled with 6 ounces sliced chicken breast, bell peppers, black olives, arugula, sun-dried tomatoes, feta cheese, and $\frac{1}{4}$ cup hummus

MEAL 3

Spaghetti squash with 4 ounces scallops and 4 ounces shrimp topped with $\frac{1}{2}$ cup garlic-infused marinara

Side of steamed peas and carrots

SNACKS

2 hard-cooked eggs

1 stick cheese

1 apple

SUNDAY

MEAL 1

Mexican scrambled eggs (3 eggs, chopped tomatoes, onions, spinach, bell peppers, $\frac{1}{2}$ cup shredded cheese, $\frac{1}{4}$ cup salsa)

1 orange

MEAL 2

Tuna melt sandwich (1 can tuna, 2 slices multigrain bread, $\frac{1}{2}$ sliced avocado, 1 slice Cheddar cheese)

MEAL 3

8 ounces Cajun-rubbed top sirloin with grilled zucchini, onion, and steamed spinach

SNACKS

1 cup cottage cheese

1 handful of almonds

YOUR 4-WEEK SIX-PACK EATING PLAN

WEEK 3

MONDAY

MEAL 1
Power protein oatmeal (½ cup oatmeal, 1–2 scoops protein powder, 1 cup berries)
1 cup almond milk

MEAL 2
Wild salmon salad (6 ounces wild salmon, arugula, romaine, cherry tomatoes, ¼ cup pecans, mandarin oranges)

MEAL 3
Chicken stir-fry (6 ounces chicken, snow peas, spinach, scallions, mushrooms, chestnuts, ¼ cup peanuts) served over ½ cup brown rice.

SNACKS
1 handful of almonds
2 ounces hard cheese
1 apple

TUESDAY

MEAL 1
Spicy omelet (3 eggs, 1 link spicy red-pepper chicken sausage, spinach, 2 mushrooms, 1 tablespoon Cheddar cheese, ½ cup salsa)
1 cup V8 juice

MEAL 2
Portobello mushroom and salmon kebabs mixed with onions and red, yellow, and green bell peppers
Steamed kale and cauliflower

MEAL 3
8 ounces broiled flank steak
Mixed salad with baby spinach, carrots, cucumber, radish, and sprouts

SNACKS
Protein pudding (1 tablespoon almond butter, 1 scoop protein powder, and 3 ounces almond milk; freeze for 1 hour and serve)
1 banana

WEDNESDAY

MEAL 1
Strawberry-Banana Protein Smoothie (Blend 1 banana, ½ cup strawberries, 1 cup almond milk, 1½ scoops vanilla whey protein powder, and 4 ice cubes.)

MEAL 2
Chicken spinach Parmesan (6 ounces chicken breast, 1 tablespoon Parmesan cheese, 1 clove garlic, ¼ cup marinara sauce, spinach)
Side of ½ cup quinoa

MEAL 3
8 ounces grilled steak with chimichurri sauce (1 tablespoon water, 2 tablespoons red wine vinegar, 2 minced cloves garlic, 1 teaspoon salt, ground red pepper, black pepper, olive oil)

SNACKS
1½ cups grapes
1 slice mozzarella cheese
3 ounces ham, sliced

THURSDAY

MEAL 1
Spinach, mushroom, and cheese omelet (3 eggs, 1 teaspoon salt, 1 teaspoon black pepper, ¼ cup Cheddar-Jack cheese, spinach, mushrooms)

MEAL 2
Turkey melt (6 ounces sliced turkey breast, 2 slices sprouted grain bread, 1 slice cheese, 1 teaspoon ground red pepper, tomato, lettuce, chopped celery)

MEAL 3
Chicken fajitas (8 ounces grilled, sliced chicken marinated in Cajun seasoning, ½ cup black beans, ½ cup salsa, ½ avocado, and a small flour tortilla)

SNACKS
1 cup cottage cheese
1 cup sliced strawberries

FRIDAY

MEAL 1
2 scrambled eggs
2 strips bacon
1 cup mixed berries (strawberries and blueberries)

MEAL 2
Romaine lettuce, 1 hard-cooked egg, 3 ounces sliced chicken, cherry tomatoes, small handful of sliced almonds, 1 teaspoon rice wine vinegar

MEAL 3
8 ounces grilled chicken sautéed in lime-butter sauce (2 limes, 1 tablespoon butter)
1 cup steamed spinach
1 cup mashed butternut squash
Steamed asparagus

SNACKS
3 ounces beef jerky
4 celery stalks with 1 tablespoon peanut butter

SATURDAY

MEAL 1
Pineapple-Banana Breeze (Blend 1–2 scoops vanilla protein powder, 6 ounces almond milk, ½ cup pineapple chunks, 1 banana, 1 teaspoon vanilla extract, and 4 ice cubes.)

MEAL 2
6 ounces grilled chicken breast, ½ avocado
Grilled asparagus and zucchini

MEAL 3
Grilled shrimp and scallops (4 ounces shrimp, 4 ounces scallops)
½ cup cooked quinoa
Steamed broccoli and carrots

SNACKS
1 stick cheese
1 handful of walnuts

SUNDAY

MEAL 1
1 cup plain Greek yogurt
1 cup fresh cherries
2 hard-cooked eggs

MEAL 2
6 ounces grass-fed burger on a bed of kale

MEAL 3
Fish tacos (8 ounces grilled halibut, 2 small corn tortillas, ¼ sliced avocado, 2 tablespoons salsa, ½ cup shredded romaine, 1 cup red and yellow bell peppers, sliced onions, ½ sliced jalapeño chile pepper)

SNACKS
Berry Bliss Smoothie (Blend 4 ounces almond milk, 4 ounces water, 1 scoop vanilla protein powder, ½ cup blueberries, ½ cup strawberries, ¼ cup blackberries, and 4 ice cubes.)

**YOUR 4-WEEK
SIX-PACK
EATING PLAN**

WEEK 4

MONDAY

MEAL 1
2 ounces smoked salmon and 2 scrambled eggs on spelt toast (Lay the smoked salmon on the toasted bread and top with the scrambled eggs. Finish with your choice of red onion, capers, dill, or a squeeze of lemon.)

MEAL 2
6 ounces sesame-crusted ahi tuna served over a bed of mixed greens, drizzled with balsamic vinaigrette

MEAL 3
6–8 ounces Cajun-rubbed top sirloin with grilled zucchini, onion, and steamed spinach

SNACKS
1 banana and 1 tablespoon almond butter

2–3 hard-cooked eggs

TUESDAY

MEAL 1
Strawberry-Banana Protein Smoothie (Blend 1 banana, $\frac{1}{2}$ cup strawberries, 1 cup almond milk, $1\frac{1}{2}$ scoops vanilla whey protein powder, and 4 ice cubes.)

MEAL 2
6 ounces baked salmon with peach-mango salsa

1 cup sliced cantaloupe

Steamed spinach

MEAL 3
6–8 ounces grilled chicken breast, cooked in olive oil, topped with $\frac{1}{2}$ avocado

Side of grilled asparagus and squash

SNACKS
1 apple

3 ounces hard cheese

WEDNESDAY

MEAL 1
Mexican scrambled eggs (3 eggs, chopped tomatoes, onions, spinach, bell pepper, $\frac{1}{2}$ cup shredded cheese, $\frac{1}{4}$ cup salsa)

1 orange

MEAL 2
$\frac{1}{2}$ cup shirataki noodles with 6 ounces ground turkey, roasted spinach, and mushrooms

MEAL 3
Kebabs with 2 ounces shrimp, 6 ounces chicken, onion, and red and green bell pepper

Kale salad topped with $\frac{1}{2}$ avocado

SNACKS
1 cup cottage cheese

1 handful of almonds

THURSDAY

MEAL 1

- $1/2$ cup oatmeal, cinnamon, $1/4$ cup raisins
- 2–3 links chicken sausage

MEAL 2

- Soba noodle chicken pad thai ($1/4$ cup soba noodles, 6 ounces chicken, peas, carrots, water chestnuts, and $1/4$ cup diced peanuts. Add a sauce of 2 teaspoons sriracha and 2 tablespoons soy sauce when finished cooking.)

MEAL 3

- 4 ounces grilled calamari and 4 ounces grilled shrimp served over sautéed Swiss chard and shallots

SNACKS

- 4 strips beef jerky
- $1/4$ cup quinoa

FRIDAY

MEAL 1

- Breakfast burrito (3 eggs scrambled, 1 whole grain tortilla, shredded mozzarella cheese, 2 ounces shredded chicken, sliced tomato, onions, bell pepper, avocado)

MEAL 2

- 6 ounces roasted halibut with $1/2$ cup fava beans, yellow squash, and shallot sauce

MEAL 3

- Spicy beef and chicken stir-fry (4 ounces lean steak, 4 ounces chicken, spinach, bell peppers, onions, mushrooms, snap peas, bean sprouts, 2 tablespoons soy sauce, and as much sriracha as desired)

SNACKS

- 1 apple and 1 tablespoon almond butter
- 1 cup milk

SATURDAY

MEAL 1

- Protein Berry Smoothie (Blend 2 scoops vanilla protein powder, 6 ounces almond milk, $1/2$ cup strawberries, $1/2$ cup blueberries, $1/4$ cup blackberries, 1 tablespoon chia seeds, 1 cup spinach, and 4 ice cubes.)

MEAL 2

- Spinach wrap filled with 6 ounces sliced chicken breast, bell pepper, black olives, arugula, sun-dried tomatoes, feta cheese, and $1/4$ cup hummus

MEAL 3

- Spaghetti squash with 4 ounces scallops and 4 ounces shrimp topped with $1/2$ cup garlic-infused marinara
- Side of steamed peas and carrots

SNACKS

- 2 hard-cooked eggs
- 1 stick cheese
- 1 apple

SUNDAY

MEAL 1

- Mexican scrambled eggs (3 eggs, chopped tomatoes, onions, spinach, bell peppers, $1/2$ cup shredded cheese, $1/4$ cup salsa)
- 1 orange

MEAL 2

- Tuna melt sandwich (1 can tuna, 2 slices mulligrain bread, $1/2$ sliced avocado, 1 slice Cheddar cheese)

MEAL 3

- 8 ounces Cajun-rubbed top sirloin with grilled zucchini, onion, and steamed spinach

SNACKS

- 1 cup cottage cheese
- 1 handful of almonds

CHAPTER 19

THE WORLD'S GREATEST ABS WORKOUT

Yes, you have abs—they just need to be uncovered. And the most effective way to torch fat above your belt is by building more total body muscle, which in turn will stoke your metabolism.

The compound exercises in this plan—squats and deadlifts—not only stimulate strength gains but also train your trunk muscles harder than many traditional core exercises do, according to researchers at Appalachian State University. As a result, you'll build a leaner, stronger midsection, all without doing a single ab exercise. Not ready to give up your crunches? Set a timer for 5 minutes after you've completed all the exercises in this plan, and then finish your workout with your favorite ab moves.

WORKOUT A

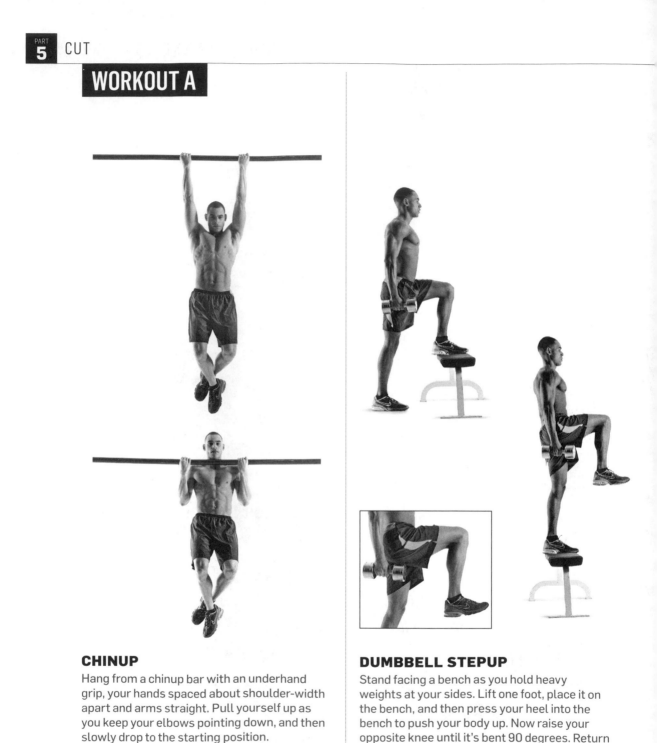

CHINUP

Hang from a chinup bar with an underhand grip, your hands spaced about shoulder-width apart and arms straight. Pull yourself up as you keep your elbows pointing down, and then slowly drop to the starting position.

Make sure your chin goes above the bar in each repetition.

DUMBBELL STEPUP

Stand facing a bench as you hold heavy weights at your sides. Lift one foot, place it on the bench, and then press your heel into the bench to push your body up. Now raise your opposite knee until it's bent 90 degrees. Return to the starting position.

Straighten your weight-bearing leg.

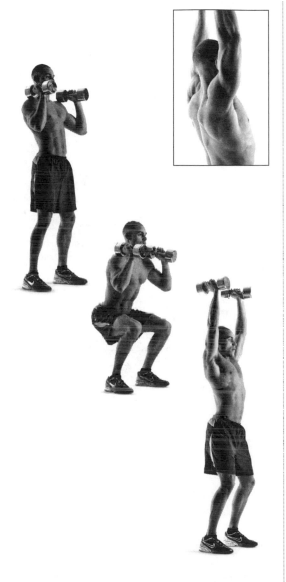

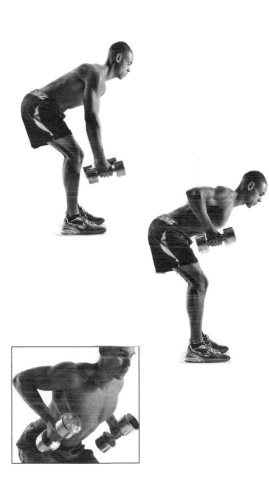

DUMBBELL SQUAT TO PRESS

Stand holding dumbbells at your shoulders with your palms facing each other. Lower yourself into a squat until your thighs are at least parallel to the floor. Push back up and press the weights overhead. Return to the starting position.

Try to keep your arms in line with your ears.

DUMBBELL ROW

Stand holding a pair of dumbbells at your sides with a neutral grip (palms facing each other). Bend forward at the waist until your back is almost parallel to the floor. Pull the weights up to your rib cage, and then lower them back down. Bend forward only to a point that will preserve the natural arch in your back.

WORKOUT B

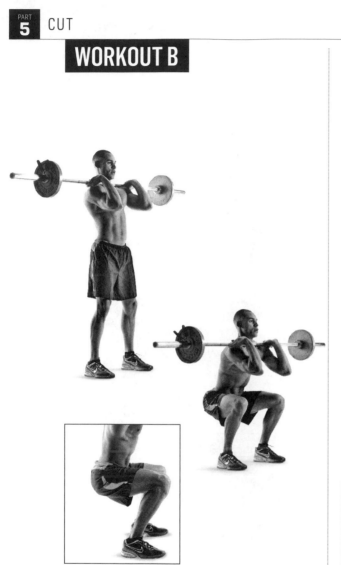

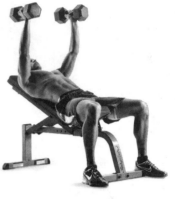

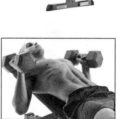

BARBELL FRONT SQUAT

Stand holding a bar with an overhand grip. Bring your elbows forward so the bar rests across the front of your shoulders with your palms up and elbows high. Lower your body and then press back to a standing position. Your upper thighs should be parallel to the floor or lower at the bottom of the move.

DUMBBELL INCLINE BENCH PRESS

Lie faceup on an incline bench with your feet flat on the floor. Hold a pair of dumbbells above your chest with straight arms, palms facing each other. Slowly lower the weights to the sides of your chest. Pause, and then push them back up. Bring the weights all the way down to the sides of your chest.

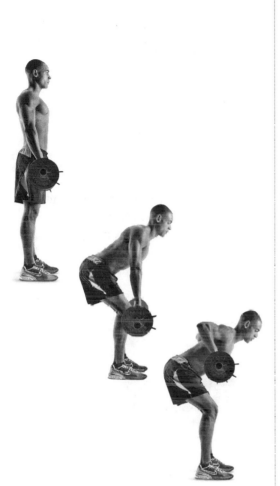

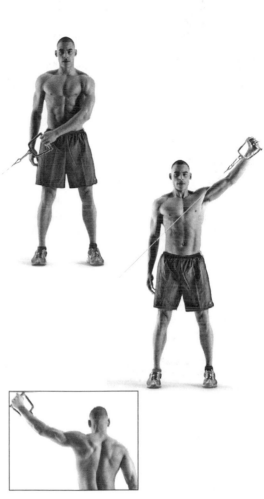

BARBELL ROMANIAN DEADLIFT TO ROW

Stand holding a barbell in front of your thighs. Keeping your knees slightly bent and your back arched, push your hips back to lower the bar to your shins. At the bottom, draw it up toward your rib cage, lower it, and then return to the starting position. Pull the bar up until your elbows pass your torso.

CABLE PNF

Stand to the left of a cable station. Grab a low-pulley cable handle with your left hand. Pull it up and across your body so that at the top of the move your palm faces forward. Reverse the path. Finish a set before repeating with your other arm. At the top, your arm should be straight and to the left of your shoulder.

YOUR 6-WEEK PLAN FOR A SIX-PACK

DIRECTIONS

Lift weights 3 days a week, alternating between the two routines described above and resting at least a day between sessions. For example, if you do workout A on Monday and Friday and workout B on Wednesday of this week, then schedule workout B for Monday and Friday and workout A for Wednesday of next week.

WEEKS 1 TO 3

Start with 5 sets of 5 repetitions of the first exercise—either the chinup or barbell front squat. Rest 2 minutes between sets. Then do the next three movements in your routine as a circuit, completing just 1 set for each exercise before progressing to the next move. Do 8 to 10 reps of each movement in the circuit, resting 60 seconds between sets. Repeat for a total of 3 rounds.

WEEKS 4 TO 6

In each workout, perform 6 sets of 3 reps for the first exercise, resting 2 to 3 minutes between sets. Then do the next three exercises as a circuit, just as you did during weeks 1 to 3—except you'll be completing 10 to 12 reps of each exercise and resting 60 seconds between moves. Do a total of 4 rounds.

Accelerate for Abs

Run off extra pounds by following this interval-training plan twice a week. Run, rest, and repeat according to the schedule below, preferably on days when you don't lift weights. You can also cycle, run stairs, or use the cardio machine of your choice.

	MAX-EFFORT SPRINT	RECOVERY	REPS
WEEK 1			
Day 1	60 seconds	180 seconds	3
Day 2	60 seconds	120 seconds	4
WEEK 2			
Day 1	60 seconds	180 seconds	4
Day 2	60 seconds	120 seconds	5
WEEK 3			
Day 1	60 seconds	180 seconds	5
Day 2	60 seconds	120 seconds	6
WEEK 4			
Day 1	60 seconds	60 seconds	5
Day 2	120 seconds	120 seconds	3
WEEK 5			
Day 1	60 seconds	60 seconds	6
Day 2	120 seconds	120 seconds	4
WEEK 6			
Day 1	60 seconds	60 seconds	7
Day 2	120 seconds	120 seconds	5

CHAPTER 20

THE NO-CRUNCH CORE EXPRESS

Ab training is easy; core training is hard. An exercise like the crunch works a tiny amount of muscle through a minuscule range of motion. Core training works your abdominal muscles along with your lower back and draws in your glutes, hamstrings, and everything in between. Even your lats are involved; the connective tissue at the bottom of your lats play a crucial role in stabilizing your spine and helping transfer force between the muscles in your upper and lower body when you row, climb, or pull.

Training that much muscle at once burns a lot of calories, even if you're not moving.

Here's an example: Assume a pushup position, with your arms straight. Lift your right arm and left leg simultaneously, and hold that position. Concentrate on keeping your body still—don't let your hips drop or your torso rotate. Keep holding. A little longer. Wait . . . okay, you lost it. No problem. Just repeat by lifting your left arm and right leg. And hold that.

Unless you're a recreational acrobat, you're probably sweating, shaking, and wheezing like an asthmatic at a Snoop Dogg concert. Train like that for 10 minutes each time you go to the gym, and it's hard not to get lean.

BUILD MUSCLE WHERE IT MATTERS

If your goal was to build your biceps, you'd target those muscles with curls. Why curls? Because you can feel your biceps contracting on each rep. Most guys use the same logic in pursuit of abs: Crunches shorten the muscles, so that must be the best way to work them.

Except it isn't.

A 2008 study in the *Journal of Strength and Conditioning Research* shows that exercises that extend your body while keeping your lower back in a safe, neutral position work the rectus abdominis—the six-pack muscle—25 percent harder than crunches do.

Try this: Grab a Swiss ball and assume a plank position—your toes on the floor and body straight from neck to ankles—but with your forearms on the ball. Slowly push the ball out and away. Go as far as you can while keeping your lower back completely stiff—that is, the arch in your lower back shouldn't increase or decrease. Pull the ball back, and repeat. Chances are, it'll take a few workouts before you can do 10 reps with a good range of motion. And you may find yourself with sore abs a day or two afterward. But at least you'll know you're truly developing these muscles.

WIN THE GAME OF LIFE

Core training isn't the answer to every fitness question. When researchers try to correlate core stability with athletic performance, the results are underwhelming. But good strength coaches include core training in their programs anyway; they know it's important for back injury prevention, if nothing else.

However, when a Canadian research team looked at specific tests of fitness and longevity, they found that men who scored lowest for abdominal endurance had more than double the risk of death from any cause over the course of the study compared with those who scored highest.

Why? The same reason strength coaches stress core training, even if it's not directly linked to goals or touchdowns. Stability of your lower back depends on the endurance of the supporting muscles. Spinal instability leads to injury. Injury can be a career killer for an athlete, and just plain deadly for an older adult.

Train your abs now and you'll have many more years to enjoy the benefits.

Three Sneaky Ways to Train Your Core

You can turn almost any exercise into one that improves core strength and stability.

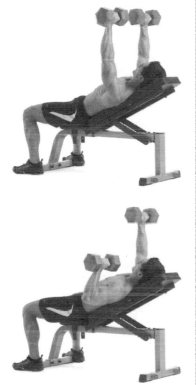

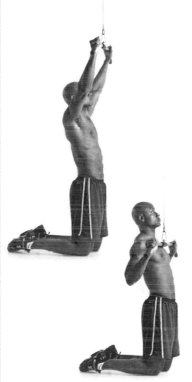

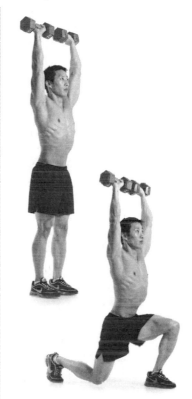

ALTERNATING DUMBBELL BENCH PRESS

Set a bench to a slight incline. Hold a pair of dumbbells straight above your shoulders. Instead of pressing both dumbells at once, lift them one at a time, in an alternating fashion. This increases core activation because you're continually changing the weight distribution on each side of your body.

KNEELING LAT PULLDOWN

Attach a triangle handle to a high pulley cable, kneel down, and pull the handle to your chest.

INTENSIFY: Perform the exercise while standing. Standing up forces your lats, lower back, and glutes to work together to stabilize your spine and pelvis.

OVERHEAD REVERSE DUMBBELL LUNGE

Hold a pair of dumbbells straight over your head. Step back with your left leg into a lunge, and return to the starting position. Do all your reps, switch sides, and repeat. Holding the weight high forces your lats and abdominals to stabilize your spine.

THE NO-CRUNCH CORE EXPRESS

If you think doing crunches, crunches, and more crunches is the best way to build your abs, prepare to be enlightened. Every exercise in this routine from Lou Schuler and Alwyn Cosgrove, C.S.C.S., coauthors of *The New Rules of Lifting for Abs*, strengthens your core—yet you won't find a single crunch. Or side bend. Or situp. What you will discover is the most effective way to train your abs from every single angle while burning off the fat that hides them. There's nothing complicated. In fact, revealing your abs has never been simpler.

DIRECTIONS

Perform this total-body workout 3 days a week, but be sure to rest at least 1 day between each session. This workout is separated into two sections: core and strength. Use the directions below each exercise, making sure you perform the core exercises first before moving on to complete the 2 strength supersets.

CORE WORKOUT

Do the exercises in the order shown, completing all the prescribed sets of each exercise before moving on to the next.

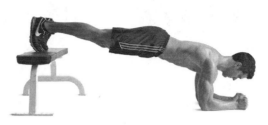

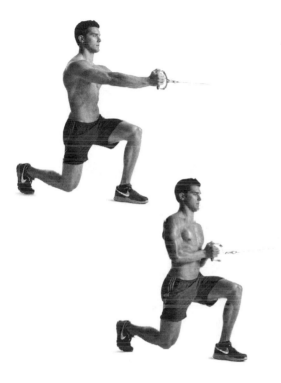

1. HALF-KNEELING CABLE CORE PRESS

Complete 1 set, holding for 30 seconds each side. Attach a D-handle at chest height to a cable machine. Kneel alongside the machine with one knee (the knee closest to the machine) bent 90 degrees and the other knee on the floor. Grab the handle with both hands, hold it in front of your chest, and brace your abs. Slowly press your arms in front of you until they're straight, hold without letting your body rotate, and bring them back to your chest. Reverse legs and and work your other side.

2. ELEVATED-FEET PLANK

Complete 10 sets, holding each set for 10 seconds followed by 10 seconds of rest. Place your feet on a bench and assume a pushup position; bend your elbows and rest your weight on your forearms instead of your hands. Your body should form a straight line from shoulders to ankles. Contract your abs as If you were about to be punched. Hold this position for the recommended time.

Your elbows should be directly below your shoulders.

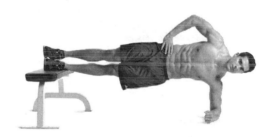

3. ELEVATED-FEET SIDE PLANK

Complete 5 sets on each side, holding for 10 seconds. Alternate back and forth until you've finished all the sets.

Lie on your left side with your legs straight. Place your feet on a bench, and prop your upper body on your left elbow and forearm. Raise your hips so your body forms a straight line from ankles to shoulders. Brace your core by contracting your abs. Hold this position for the recommended time. Then turn around so you're lying on your right side and repeat.

Make sure you maintain a straight line, not letting your hips sag.

STRENGTH WORKOUT

Do 1 set of 12 reps of exercise 1A, and rest for 45 seconds. Then do 1 set of 12 reps of exercise 1B and rest for another 45 seconds. Repeat until you've completed 3 sets of each exercise. Then move on to exercises 2A and 2B and follow the same instructions.

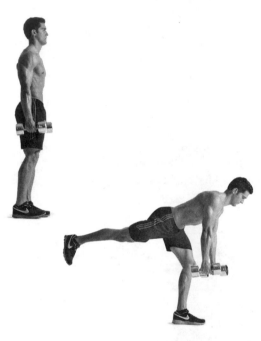

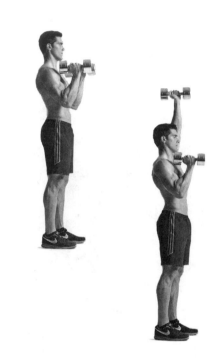

1A. SINGLE-LEG DUMBBELL STRAIGHT-LEG DEADLIFT

Using an overhand grip, hold a pair of dumbbells at arm's length next to your sides. Stand with your feet hip-width apart and your knees slightly bent. Raise your right foot off the floor and, without changing the bend in your left knee, bend at your hips and lower your torso until it's almost parallel to the floor. Pause, and return to the starting position. Do all your reps, switch legs, and repeat.

Your raised leg should stay in line with your body.

1B. ALTERNATING DUMBBELL OVERHEAD PRESS

Hold a pair of dumbbells just outside your shoulders, your arms bent and palms facing each other. Set your feet at shoulder-width and bend your knees slightly. Press each dumbbell up, one at a time, until your arm is straight. As you lower one dumbbell, press the other one up, in an alternating fashion.

Keep your arm in line with your torso as you press the weight above your head.

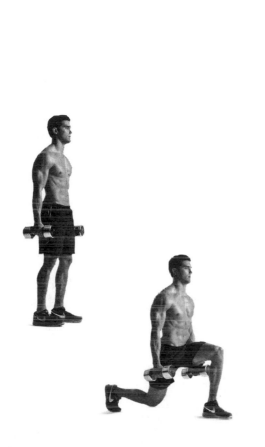

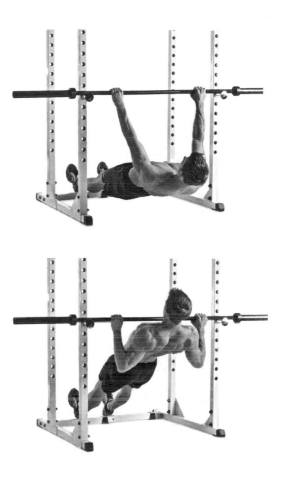

2A. REVERSE DUMBBELL LUNGE

Hold a pair of dumbbells at arm's length next to your sides, your palms facing each other. Step backward with your right leg. Then lower your body until your front knee is bent at least 90 degrees. Pause, and push yourself back to the starting position. Do all your reps, switch legs, and repeat.

Pull your shoulders back and stand as tall as you can.

2B. INVERTED ROW

Using an overhand, shoulder-width grip, grab a bar that's been secured at about waist height. Hang with your arms completely straight, hands positioned directly above your shoulders, and heels touching the floor. Your body should form a straight line from your ankles to your head. Pull your shoulder blades back, and continue to pull with your arms to lift your chest to the bar. Pause, and lower your body back to the starting position.

Keep your body rigid through the entire movement.

INDEX

Boldface page references indicate illustrations or photographs. Underscored references indicate boxed text.